Baby Dreams

Baby Dreams

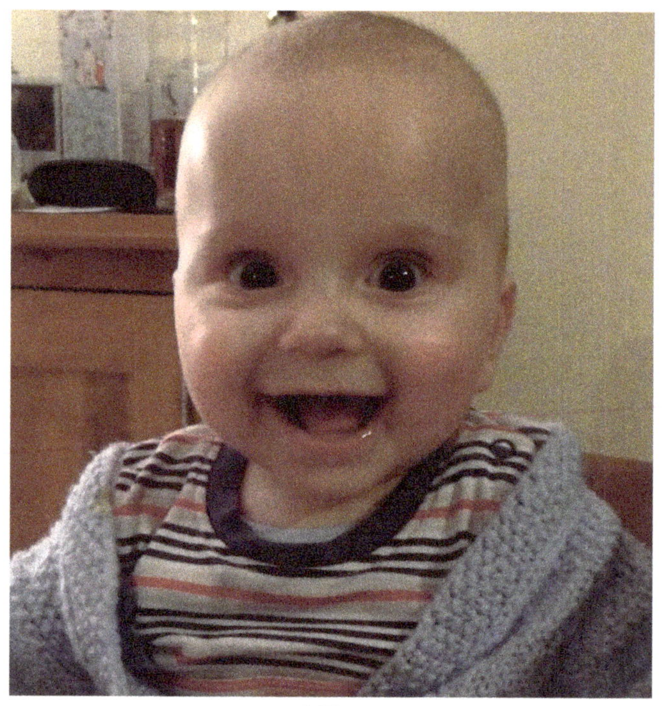

William

Baby Dreams

LOUISE WARNEFORD

Published by New Generation Publishing in 2019

Copyright © Louise Warneford 2019

The author asserts the moral right under the
Copyright, Designs and Patents Act 1988 to be
identified as the author of this work.

All Rights reserved. No part of this publication may
be reproduced, stored in a retrieval system or
transmitted, in any form or by any means without the
prior consent of the author, nor be otherwise circulated
in any form of binding or cover other than that which
it is published and without a similar condition being
imposed on the subsequent purchaser.

ISBN: 978-1-78955-436-6

www.newgeneration-publishing.com

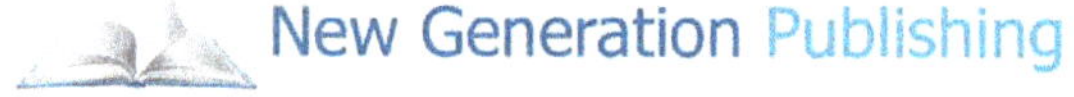
New Generation Publishing

Come on, we gotta keep the light burning
Come on, we gotta keep on dreaming.

From 'Dream Baby Dream', by Bruce Springsteen

PREFACE

This is the story of how, after 18 miscarriages and years of heartache and despair, I finally achieved my overwhelming desire to become a mother. I make no claim to offer any medical advice regarding repeat miscarriages, only to show what worked for me. If you have been unable to carry a baby to full-term, my dearest wish now is that the same treatment will work for you too.

CHAPTER ONE

If I had known my odds of carrying a baby to full-term, I think I would have thrown in my cards at the start. But had I done this, William Oliver Warneford would not be in the world, and it would be a less joyful place.

Without William, I would not have written this book. Without William, I'm not even sure I would still be here, and I don't say that lightly. But when life is kicking you hard and relentlessly it's understandable to want to escape the pain, forever. My maternal grandmother, Leah Riley, used to say, "The Lord will only dish it out to those who can take it", but even her faith may have been shaken had she been alive during the trauma of my recurrent miscarriage. Now, though, I think she was probably right in her belief.

Nanny Riley was right about a lot of things, and it was to her that my sister Julie and I often used to turn for help and advice. She was like a second mother and we spent a lot of time at her home, including most weekends. The fact that she was a much better cook than our mum added to her appeal. Nanny Riley was one of the oldest siblings in a very big family and had to help bring up the younger ones, giving her an obvious head-start in how to care for children. She and Grandad Joe ensured their children – Gwen (my mother), Ed and Bob – had a stable childhood. Grandad worked as an RAF medic during the war, then as a boiler engineer. He was very good at art and we used to get him to draw us pictures for Halloween and Christmas. He died when I was six.

I'd like to say that Nanny Riley passed her common sense on to my mother, but it wouldn't be true – Mum was as crazy as a box of frogs. It's difficult to describe exactly why this was but I think it came down to an absence of logic. For example, she would always buy my clothes three sizes too big so that I could 'grow into them', but, unsurprisingly, they always wore out before then. Something else totally bonkers that she used to do was put the leftovers from the weekly Sunday roast in the twin-tub so that it wouldn't be picked at by greedy little fingers and could be used to make a meal the following day.

Although Mum may not have inherited Nanny Riley's practicality and sensibleness, she did share the same great intuition. In some ways this appeared almost as a sixth sense, but it was more the ability to understand someone's true nature, which I suppose is all tied up with strong natural empathy. My mum would do anything for anyone, including giving you her last penny if she thought you needed it more than she did.

My dad is intelligent and knowledgeable about a lot of

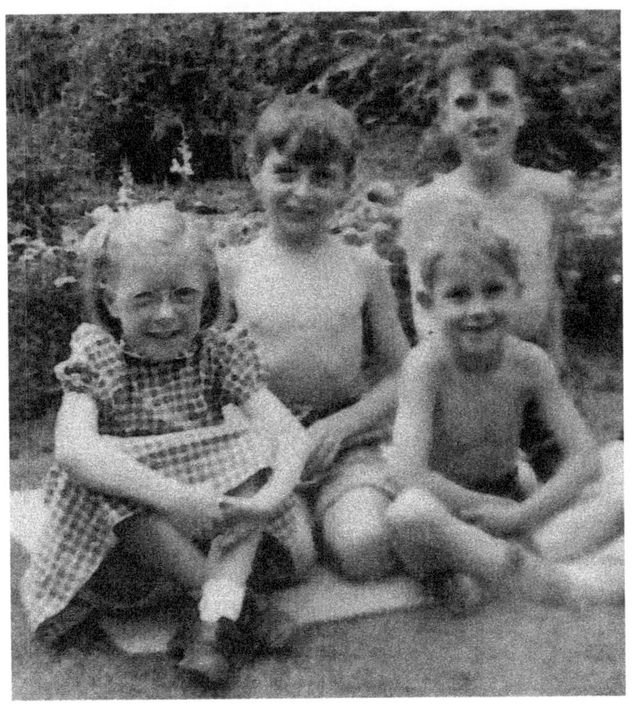

Mum, Cousin Eric, Bob and Ed

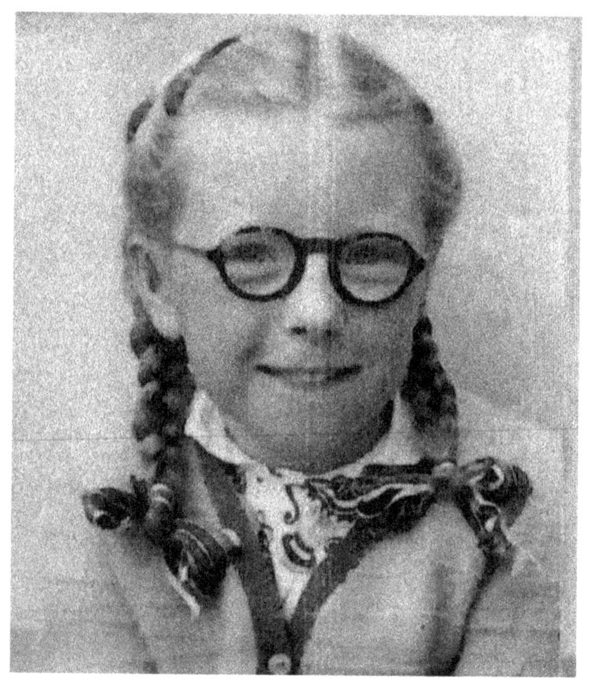

Mum, around 1950

things, e.g. history (he knows everything about the Second World War!), but he also has some rather odd ways. I remember how horrified I was when I saw my first bicycle, which he had just dragged out of the Manchester Ship Canal, covered in rust and gunk. But he did it up so beautifully that all the local kids wanted to have a go on it. He also made my sister and me a snow sledge, which was great fun but wouldn't have passed any safety test. Unfortunately, his attempt at making a kite did not have the same success. It consisted of brown paper and a thin wooden edging, which I think was bamboo, and it may not have flown but it certainly looked good. I'm sure now that Mum and Dad knew it would never fly but were just trying to keep us occupied.

Dad's way of teaching me to ride my bike was also unconventional – no stabilisers for little Louise, instead I was given a push down the road and had to learn instantly. His attitude to me falling off was, 'Well, you won't do it again, will you?'. Being taught to swim by my father was also an unnerving experience – thrown in the deep end, where I either sank or swam. This may seem very harsh but, of course, he would not have left me to drown, and although I'm not a strong swimmer, his system worked.

Despite my parents' oddities, I had a genuinely happy childhood. Although we could never afford to go to Butlins or Pontins – the dream destination then for many children – we went camping or caravanning every year, usually to Black Rock Sands in North Wales, Scarborough or Bude. Whenever we went camping, our Mum always fed us soup over mashed potato or over pork pie – urgh. On one holiday, when my sister and I were fighting over a ball, my dad's solution to the argument was to fetch a knife from the caravan kitchen and cut the ball in half!

I think it was these holidays that sparked my love for the outdoors, especially hill walking. Although I also enjoy low-level hikes, hill walking can give you a stronger sense of achievement. We've particularly enjoyed following Wainwright's walks, and we have also hiked up Snowdon and Ben Nevis. Dad used to take Julie and me out for walks at home too, sometimes just to give Mum a break. And we were often dragged around

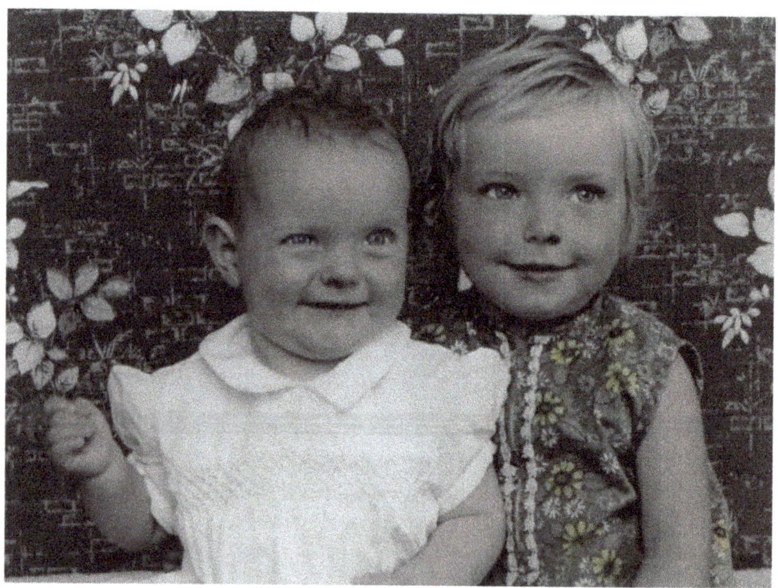

Left to right: me and Julie

museums, which I didn't particularly enjoy; they were nowhere near as interesting for children as many museums are now, with their interactive displays, etc.

Julie and I were also lucky as children to have pets, golden Labradors. First there was Kip, who was followed by Ben. We got Ben when I was seven and he died when I was 22. Another example of my mum's craziness was that she used to cook a dinner for our dogs every day too – pork chops, sausage and mash, fish and chips... I remember one Christmas my sister and I felt so sorry for Ben not having proper dog food that we pooled our pocket money and bought him a tin of Pal.

Like most people, my personality was shaped by inherited characteristics, the daily influence of my parents, and my environment, although, of course, I would not have been aware of this as I was growing up. I was born in Clatterbridge Hospital, Birkenhead on 1st November 1967, almost two years after Julie, and grew up in Ellesmere Port. Mum stayed at home to look after us until we started school, then she worked as a cleaner and waitress. Dad was a steel rigger and his contracts took him away from home a lot. He later worked at the docks in Eastham as a ships' rigger.

Dad's mother, Dolly, had him at 16. His father, Joseph Bryde, was killed in 1942 when the motor tanker he was serving on, British Resource, was torpedoed off Bermuda. Being widowed so young, and without any safety net of benefits to fall back on in those days, my grandmother was forced to put Dad into care. He was placed in Torpenhow

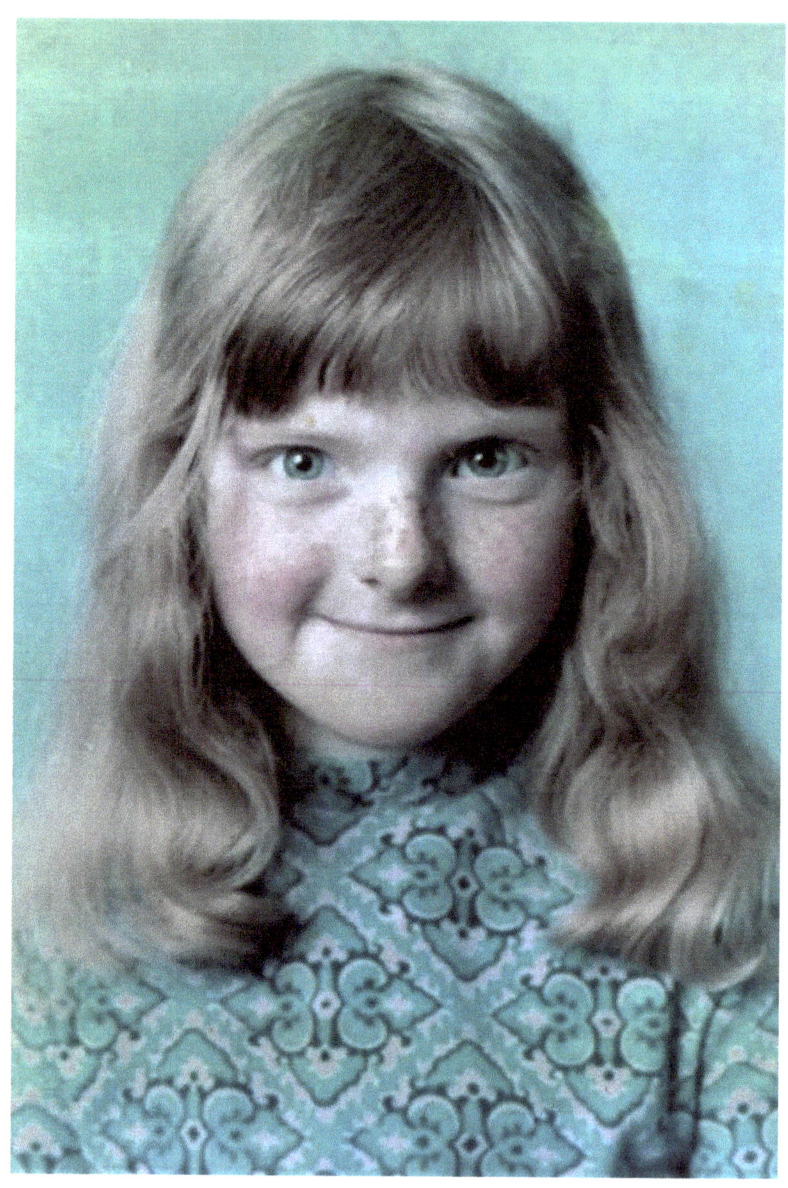

Me, primary school

Open Air School on the Wirral and remembers being there in 1953 when Edmund Hillary and Sherpa Tenzing conquered Mount Everest and during the Queen's Coronation. I would never judge my grandmother for passing Dad into the care of others – she was basically a good person but was in a very difficult position. She later remarried, and about eight years after my dad was born she had another child, Carol. But this marriage ended in divorce, either when she was pregnant with Carol or soon after her birth, I'm not sure. It wasn't long before she got married again, for the last time, to Bob Draper, so Julie and I always called her Nanny Draper. She took Dad back intermittently, which is how she came to have a presence in my life. I don't know how long Dad stayed with her at any one time, or the reasons for him being put back into care, but it all had an obvious impact on their relationship and they were never very close as a result. Dad and his sister, though, have a strong bond.

So, my father definitely suffered neglect as a child, which was no doubt responsible for some of his behaviour as an adult. Apart from the unusual parenting methods mentioned previously, he could be quite moody and had an explosive temper. Even though he always calmed down quickly after his outbursts, they did affect my mother's nerves. Mum and Dad still loved each other, though, and they both had hearts of gold; there was never any shortage of affection in our home. When Mum died, her death hit my father very hard. Dad is 76 now and still lives in Ellesmere Port. Unfortunately, his health is not good, with heart problems, COPD and fibromyalgia. I try to visit him as often as possible, to help take the load off my sister. Carol is also a huge support to him.

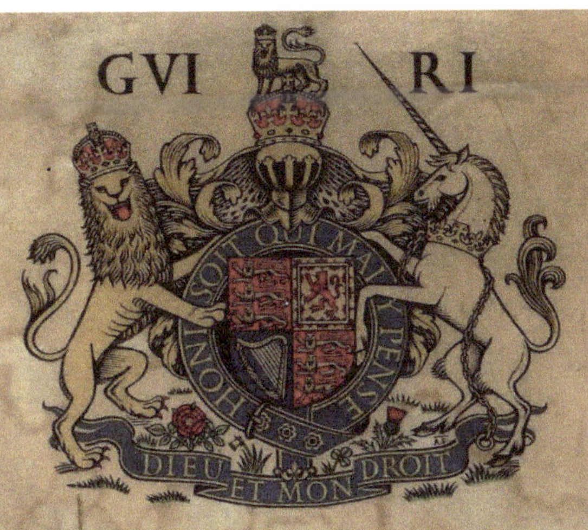

Honour certificate for my paternal grandfather, Joseph Bryde

I left school at 16 and then studied community care at college. After this, I found hotel work in the Lake District. Although I enjoyed my employment there, after a couple of years I felt it was time to move on. My decision to join the Navy, Army and Air Force Institutes (NAAFI) as a catering assistant was inspired by the opportunity it offered to work abroad. For my first year, I was based at Ternhill in Shropshire. Although my first posting was to RAF Valley, in Anglesey, the rest of my NAAFI work was in army camps.

The time I spent with the NAAFI in Germany was particularly enjoyable, with so much camaraderie between us all that it felt as if we were one big family. It was also in Germany that I met a lovely man, Andy, who was serving in the British Army. Before meeting him, my relationship experiences had not been good, with my first boyfriend being both physically and mentally abusive towards me, and the other two unfaithful. After having my confidence in the ability to judge a person's true character dented, Andy showed me that there were good men in the world, and I grew to love him very much. But after four or five years as a couple, he was posted to Hong Kong. Although we tried hard to stay together, it was just too difficult, and after a while he met someone else. I was extremely upset when we split up. I know it's futile to dwell on the 'what ifs' but I have often wondered if things might have been better for me if I'd tried to have a child with Andy. I don't mean this as a way of holding on to him through ties of fatherhood, rather that my fertility problems would have come to light earlier and, with the right treatment, I might have been able to have a baby sooner.

Then, after seven years in the NAAFI and ascending as far as possible within its ranks, I knew I needed a new challenge. So, I made the decision to leave Germany and return to the UK to train as an air steward.

I soon learned that there is no real glamour attached to being cabin crew. Yes, you get to visit interesting countries, but never for long. And being on your feet all the time, working non-stop during long flights, is exhausting. The responsibility attached to the job is huge, with the safety of the passengers being the ultimate priority. So, I never at any stage allowed my personal worries to influence my decision making while at work. It was this professionalism that enabled me to deal with an emergency landing, where I oversaw the chute evacuation of over 80 passengers in 60 seconds. The fact that I was so committed to my job and always worked to the very best of my

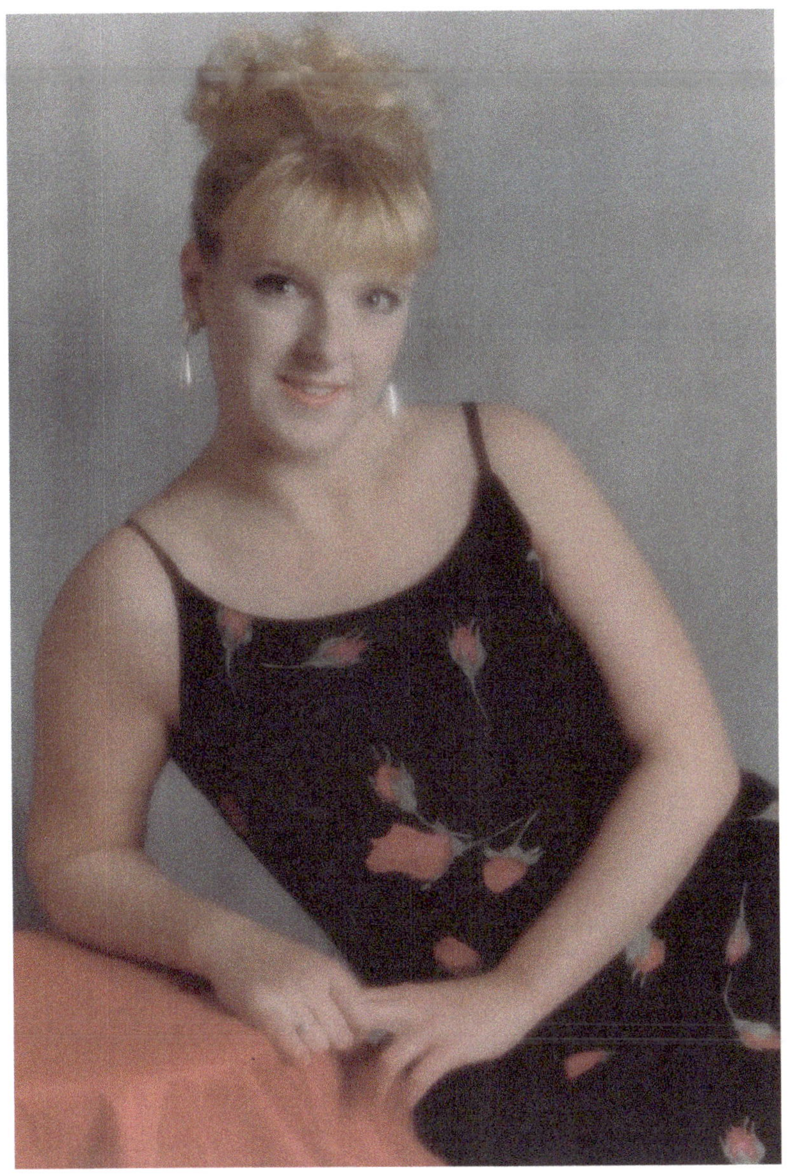

Me, in my 20s

ability will always be something of which I am proud.

Around March 1999, as I was waiting at the airport for a flight, a tall, blond, blue-eyed stranger walked into the cabin-crew staff area. It was just me in there, having a cuppa and reading through some paperwork. As he came through the door, I said "Hi" and then quickly looked back down at what I'd been reading. As a very chatty person, it would have been the most natural thing in the world for me to strike up a conversation, but I was suddenly too shy. Fortunately, he felt no such nerves.

"Mind if I join you for a brew?"

Would I mind?

"Er, of course not, I'm just waiting for my flight."

He made a cup of tea, and I felt myself glancing at the chair next to me. Taking this as a cue, he sat down.

"I haven't seen you before – are you new?" He gave a friendly smile.

"Yes – you?"

"No, I'm as old as the hills, been here years." He reached over the table to shake my hand. "I'm Mark, by the way, and it's good to meet you."

"Louise, and it's nice to meet you too." So nice.

In no time at all Mark made me feel at ease and I was sorry when my flight was called and I had to say goodbye. Although we weren't to see each other again for about six months, I certainly didn't forget about him.

CHAPTER THREE

A few weeks after meeting Mark, as I drove up the M6 the traffic was heavy, rain was hitting the windscreen and I could feel the tears running down my face. I put on my favourite music, Bruce Springsteen, and tried to pull myself together. I was on my way to Clatterbridge Hospital, to be with my mother. She had a very rare cancer, of the adrenal gland, and we were going to hear her prognosis.

The old medical books in the oncologist's room gave off a strong musty odour. My wheelchair-bound mum was surrounded by me, Dad, Julie, and her two brothers, with whom she always had a strong bond. They say there's safety in numbers, but this certainly wasn't the case then. As the oncologist spoke to Mum, his words rang in my ears like a siren: "I'm sorry Mrs Bryde, but you might as well go home and enjoy your last few months with your family." I could not believe that my mother, only 55 years old, was going to die; it was unthinkable.

For the first couple of months after this traumatic meeting,

I was consumed with trying to find a cure for Mum. All that conventional medicine could offer her by this stage was palliative care. After spending time at the local library, I found a reference to an alternative/holistic treatment called the Gerson Therapy™ and set about looking into it in detail.

According to the Gerson Institute:

"The Gerson Therapy™ is a natural treatment that activates the body's extraordinary ability to heal itself through an organic, plant-based diet, raw juices, coffee enemas and natural supplements […] with no damaging side effects. This powerful, natural treatment boosts the body's own immune system to heal cancer, arthritis, heart disease, allergies, and many other degenerative diseases […]. Rather than treating only the symptoms of a particular disease, the Gerson Therapy™ treats the causes of most degenerative diseases: toxicity and nutritional deficiency.

An abundance of nutrients from copious amounts of fresh, organic juices are consumed every day, providing your body with a super-dose of enzymes, minerals and nutrients. These substances then break down diseased tissue in the body, while coffee enemas aid in eliminating toxins from the liver […]. Degenerative diseases render the body increasingly unable to excrete waste materials adequately, commonly resulting in liver and kidney failure. The Gerson Therapy™ uses intensive detoxification to eliminate wastes, regenerate the liver, reactivate the immune system and restore the body's essential defenses – enzyme, mineral and hormone systems. With generous, high-quality nutrition, increased oxygen availability, detoxification, and improved metabolism, the cells – and the body – can regenerate, become healthy and prevent future illness."

I thought this therapy must be worth a try, after all there was nothing else that could be done for Mum through the conventional medicine route. So, I took her for a consultation at the Gerson Therapy™ centre in Birkenhead. Here, she was given a programme specifically tailored to her complex medical needs, e.g. she was unable to have the coffee enemas due to liver problems. A charity that was associated with the therapy at the time lent us a juicing machine and press and also plumbed a purifier into our water supply.

All the preparation involved in following Mum's treatment meant that I didn't stop working all day long. Chopping, peeling, blitzing – everything had to be made fresh on a daily basis; no pre-preparation and chilling overnight was allowed. Although my sister agreed that we should give the therapy a try, she had just had her daughter Catherine and was unable to help as much as she would have liked. The treatment was so strict and time-consuming to administer that we weren't able to take Mum out for full-day trips, etc., which did prove to be rather a bind for us all. Despite these drawbacks, Mum felt genuinely empowered by the treatment.

Although this regime was difficult to follow, I worked through it tirelessly, hoping that a miracle would happen and Mum would beat the cancer. For almost 12 months, as soon as I landed at home after a long-haul trip, often in the middle of the night, I would drive to my parents' house to help look after her. Although, in the end, I wasn't able to save Mum, she lived a lot longer than expected and her tumour did shrink considerably.

I really believe that if the doctors had diagnosed her condition six months earlier she would have survived.

When the end came for Mum, it was unexpected. She had been having intermittent good days and bad days but had not reached the final stages of her illness (unlike Nanny Draper, for example, who had died in a hospice). It was mid-December 2000 and I was in Italy on a short break, leaving Mum in Dad and Julie's capable hands. I had rung Mum from the airport on arrival and she sounded great, telling me she had just made Dad some breakfast. Then, on the fourth day of my visit, Julie left a message on my new work mobile to say that Mum had been rushed to hospital with breathing difficulties. I flew straight home, but she died before I got there. The cause of her death was pneumonia. She had just turned 56.

Although I've never been a churchgoer, I have always believed that there is a positive force living among us, and 'God' is just a name for it. The death of my mother at such a young age reinforced this belief in another lifeforce; I just had to trust that she had gone to a 'better place'.

CHAPTER FOUR

It was about September, 1999 and the smell of stale beer hit me as I walked through the door of the airport bar. My nose was still twitching when I saw Mark on the other side of the room, leaning against the bar. At the sight of him, my spirits lifted. Although I had been impressed by him on our first meeting, now I was really smitten. His tan made his kind blue eyes even more attractive. He grinned at me and held up a bottle of Becks, to which I responded with a nod and my most enchanting smile.

That night, we talked and laughed together non-stop, which was such a relief to me after the constant anxiety I was experiencing over Mum's illness. We were oblivious to the time passing and to the others in the room. I learned that Mark had got married at a very young age, to Helen, but the marriage had not lasted long, due mainly to their youth. He then married Sue, with whom he had two daughters, May and Evie. He and Sue had been together for 12 years before recently separating.

Mark and I became close extremely quickly. We share similar thoughts, and have finished each other's sentences since very early on in our relationship. We are matched with regard to feelings, too, and are both very emotional. Because I was so sure from early on that Mark was the right man for me, I was keen for him to meet my mum and dad. When I introduced him to Mum, I could see that she liked him straightaway. Later, she patted me gently on the hand and, echoing my own thoughts, said, "He's the one for you, Louise." I'm so glad that Mark and Mum did get to meet each other.

May was six and Evie four when Mark and I first started dating and so were too young to understand that their parents would not be getting back together. I got very attached to them from the start.

Mark was always so kind, patient and understanding with May and Evie. His love for them really shone through. The more I saw of what an amazing father he was, the more my thoughts turned to the possibility of having children of our own. In the back of my mind, I had always wanted to be a mother, but being with Mark seemed to set off my maternal alarm. This desire to try for a child was not a clinical decision though; I just knew Mark and I were right for each other and that to have his baby would make everything perfect.

Ah – but life is never that simple, is it? I think it was after Mark and I had been seeing each other for about five months that I first broached the subject of us having a child together. This may sound too soon but, as I said, I had no doubts

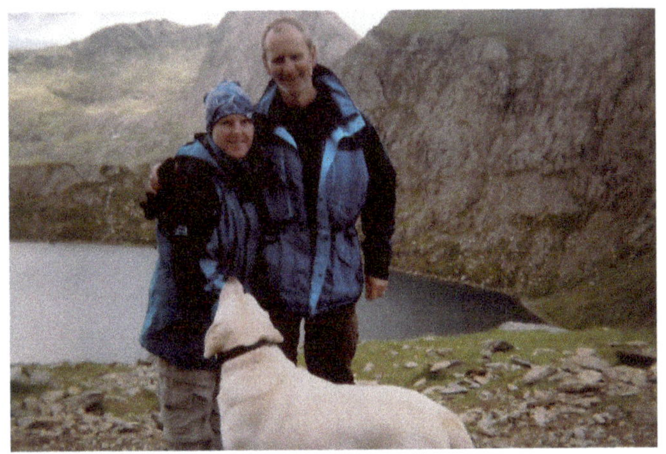

Mark and me

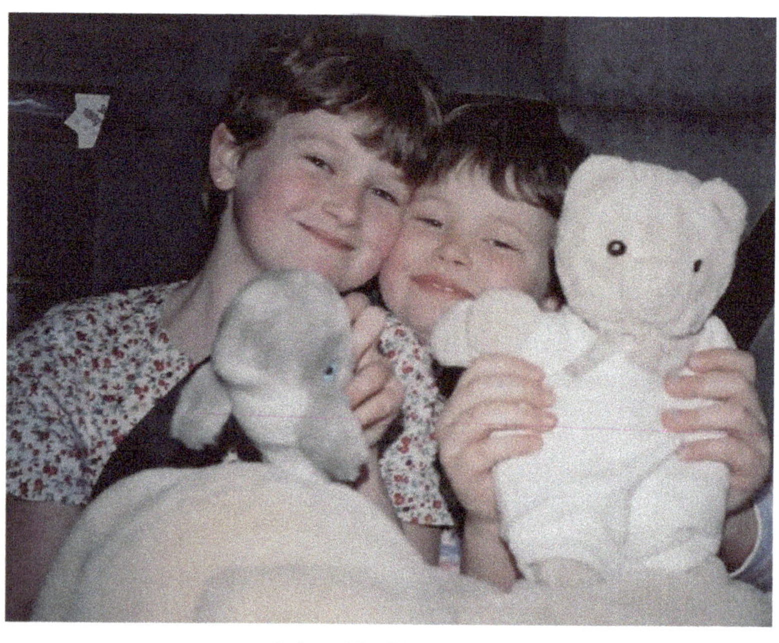

Left to right: May and Evie

about us being right for each other. I knew it would not be an easy conversation, having sensed that, at six years my senior, Mark's enthusiasm for starting all over again with a new baby would be limited. So, wanting to find the right moment for the discussion, I booked us a table at an Indian restaurant. I don't think I will ever be able to forget that evening.

I was feeling really jittery from the outset. The fact that Mark had had a vasectomy, with its obvious implications regarding fertility, made me feel particularly nervous. Sue had not wanted any more children so Mark, not imagining at the time that he and Sue would ever split up, decided to take responsibility for ensuring there were no further pregnancies. When I had learned that the man who had awakened my wish for a baby was not actually able to father any more, it had felt like a dirty trick. It was no one's fault, of course, but it was still a source of great sadness to me. So, knowing that any hope of us having a child together would involve, at the very least, Mark trying to have his vasectomy reversed really added to my anxiety.

I looked nervously around at the restaurant's soft lighting, big mirrors, pillars and chandeliers, trying to summon up the courage to tell Mark about my wish for a baby of our own. But I couldn't say it. I couldn't eat either and soon the chicken korma, my favourite curry dish, started to congeal.

Mark was enjoying his chicken madras in the same way he always did. Then he looked at me quizzically. "Not hungry, Lou?" he said.

"I think I ate too much at lunchtime," I replied, making a

swirling pattern with my fork in the slowly solidifying curry.

"Would you like me to do aeroplanes for you?" Mark laughed. "It always worked with May and Evie."

This prompted an image in my head of Mark doing zooming aerial acrobatics with a forkful of food. For our child. And then I couldn't stop myself.

"There's something I need to tell you."

Mark gulped loudly, and not because his curry was too hot. "What's wrong?"

The look of concern on his face made me realise that he either thought I was ill or I wanted to finish with him, and this made me feel even worse.

"Don't worry, nothing's wrong, at all. It's just that I've been doing a lot of thinking lately and . . ."

Mark had stopped eating now too. "And what?"

"I'd really like us to try for a baby." There, I'd said it.

For a moment or two, Mark looked at me as if I were a stranger who had just invited myself to dine at the table with him. Then he sighed so loudly I'm surprised he didn't blow out the table candle.

"You know I've had a vasectomy."

"But they can often be reversed and –"

"Lou – I had it done for a reason." Mark ran his hand through his hair. "I don't want anymore children."

Although I had anticipated that Mark would have reservations about us trying for a child of our own, his almost instant dismissal of my hopes upset me more than I could ever have imagined. I squeezed my eyelids shut in an effort to stop the tears, but it didn't work.

"Oh, Lou, come on, it's not the end of the world. You know I love you, and I think we're fine just as we are." Mark tried to give me a reassuring smile. "Aren't we?"

I couldn't answer. I knew that nothing I said would make him change his mind.

When I returned home that evening, I asked myself whether I would be able to stay with Mark now that I knew we would not be having children of our own. The fact I understood that his daughters were enough for him didn't lessen my deep need for a child of my own.

Spending time with Mark and the girls, and knowing that he would not change his mind about looking into treatment to enable me to have a child too, eventually became unbearable. For months and months, I had tried so hard to convince myself that I was happy with what I already had but my yearning for a baby was just too strong. So, although it broke my heart, I had to end our relationship.

I missed Mark, and May and Evie, dreadfully and was so unhappy. I desperately wanted this longing for a baby to disappear, so that I could get on with my life, but it was impossible. I made a great effort not to let my depression show, though, and the darkness and sadness I felt at this time was noticeable only to my sister and a couple of close friends.

Then a few months later, Mark and I met at our

headquarters' local pub. I'd had no idea he was going to be there and I think he was surprised to see me too. He said that he had missed me, and we talked and talked. The result of this long, honest conversation was a reconciliation and Mark agreeing to look into fertility treatment with me. I still loved him and was overjoyed at his change of heart. Finally, I had been given hope.

CHAPTER FIVE

Our first step was to sign up with the Oxford Fertility Unit at the John Radcliffe Hospital. The consultant explained that it would be difficult to reverse Mark's vasectomy because a lot of his tube had been removed, and the fact that it had been carried out over five years previously didn't help matters. And even if the reversal were attempted, we would have to wait 12–18 months before we could hope for Mark's sperm to show signs of life again. Also, my age was starting to work against me: the wait involved would mean I would be heading for my mid-30s by the time any hoped-for conception could take place. So, our consultant was of the opinion that the best course of action for us would be intra-uterine insemination (IUI) using donor sperm. Literature given to me by the clinic describes this process as follows:

> "Donor insemination is carried out when sperm are completely absent or if they carry a genetic disorder. Donors are carefully screened and matched to the physical characteristics of the patient. A discussion regarding the implications of donor insemination will be required with the Counsellor to ensure you are both comfortable with the use of a donor. Semen is prepared and concentrated prior to placement in the uterus using a fine catheter (intra-uterine insemination). For success, the fallopian tubes must be open. We ensure the female partner is ready to ovulate by scanning the ovaries. We then time the insemination for when the egg is predicted to have been released into the fallopian tube."

After the IUI treatment, there followed the standard two-week wait until we found out whether or not the insemination had been successful. Time can never again pass more slowly than it did during those 14 days. For me at least, there were definite stages to how I felt during this wait:

Days 1–3

This is the hopeful stage, feeling that you have done everything you possibly can and it was now all in the hands of the gods.

Day 4

You believe you're pregnant and that a little embryo is busy making a comfortable home for itself in the lining of your uterus. Your senses are so heightened that you think you can feel a difference in your body.

Day 5

After all your positive feelings, the doubt starts to kick in. You face up to the fact that you had just been imagining those changes in your body.

Day 6

You think that Google has become your new best friend. How long does it take for implantation to occur? How long does it take before the human chorionic gonadotropin (hCG) can be detected? What's the best early pregnancy-test kit on the market? You're on all the online forums about pregnancy.

Day 7

You've had enough of Google.

Days 8–9

You look at the home pregnancy tests that you've bought from Amazon and you're desperate to try one.

Day 10

You try one. And another one. And another...

Day 11

With just a few days until the official test date (OTD), your sense of anticipation is so high it's almost unbearable. You are also very aware that if the official test result is negative, you will have to relive this stress all over again.

Day 14

The test is negative. Disappointment and despair.

The clinic ensured that there was a different sperm donor for each insemination attempt and always tried to match the physical characteristics of the father. Although the following month did result in a positive pregnancy test, unfortunately it was a biochemical pregnancy. This is a pregnancy that has stopped developing before about five-and-a-half weeks. Because it has stopped growing before it is large enough to be seen with ultrasound, the only evidence that the pregnancy existed is the positive pregnancy test itself – hence the term 'biochemical'. (During my long fertility journey, I was to endure eight of these cruel biochemical pregnancies. Early on, I also had an ectopic pregnancy, where the fertilised egg implants itself outside of the womb, usually in one of the fallopian tubes. This was also a deeply upsetting experience.)

CHAPTER SIX

When Mark and I reunited and he'd agreed to look into fertility treatment, I'd been full of joy. I had found the man of my dreams and everything in my life had finally come together. The thought of ever suffering a miscarriage never entered my head. So, when the third attempt at donor-sperm fertilisation was successful but I then went on to lose the baby, I felt as if I had been hit by a bus.

Because I was under the care of the clinic, I had scans at six, eight and ten weeks, and they were all okay. Then, for my 12-week scan, I was referred to the general hospital. I was on my own as Mark was working away and we'd had no reason to suspect that anything might be wrong. I think the whole building must have heard me scream when I was told that there was "no foetal heartbeat". There is nothing on earth that can prepare you for those three words. This type of miscarriage is classed by the medical profession as a silent or missed miscarriage.

The pregnancy charity Tommy's say that one in every four women will miscarry and the chance of losing a baby increases with each miscarriage. For example, if you miscarry your first pregnancy (a chance of 5%) your chance of miscarrying again rises to 19% and if you miscarry that second time your chance of a third rises to 24%.

I was given three choices as to what to do next: take an abortion tablet; wait for the baby to come out naturally; or have a Dilation and Curettage (D&C). The latter is often performed after a first-trimester miscarriage and involves first dilating/expanding the cervix to open it and then removing the contents of the uterus by scraping the uterine lining. I chose this option as I could not bear the thought of having to go into labour when I knew that my baby was no longer alive.

The procedure was carried out at Swindon Hospital, where I was on a ward with women who were having voluntary abortions. I would never judge anyone who chooses, for whatever reason, to have an abortion and think that for most women it must be a tough decision to make. But I still found it extremely upsetting to be there, not least because of a woman in the bed next to me, who had taken an abortion tablet. With only a curtain separating us, I could obviously hear everything, could hear her excited voice: "It's the size of a grape!" This will live with me until the day I die.

Being on a ward with women undergoing voluntary abortions didn't get easier with any of my subsequent miscarriages. Another time I remember with pure horror was in hospital in Oxford. The woman in the bed opposite, waiting for her D&C, was being visited by her husband and toddler. I don't like saying this, not only because of the pain the memory still causes me but also because I don't want to appear judgemental, but it was clear that this woman was also perfectly okay about having an abortion. As she was laughing at her toddler's antics, I was in torment. I wanted to scream and beg her, "*Please, please, please* don't do this, let me have your baby instead!" Such constant, intense longing that never eases can lead even the strongest person to the brink of madness.

CHAPTER SEVEN

After losing so many IUI-treatment pregnancies, my fertility specialist recommended that we try In-vitro Fertilisation (IVF), which would have the added benefit of enabling the quality of my eggs to be evaluated. But even though the eggs turned out to be all top quality, the results with IVF were the same as with IUI – more miscarriages, more pain. The grief was unbearable.

Still, we kept on trying with IVF, for a number of years. Then, one day, I was asked to attend an appointment with my specialist. I knew that even though my eggs seemed to be of excellent quality, my specialist was nevertheless of the opinion that there was something wrong with them. So I was very apprehensive that he was going to tell me that all treatment was futile and needed to stop. But to my surprise and great relief, he suggested that I start trying donor embryos, which are used for women with complex medical problems.

The waiting list for this was long but I was so buoyed up with hope at what the procedure could mean to me that the time passed relatively quickly. When the call came to tell me that a donor was available, I felt a tingle of joy. But it was all to no avail – I kept on losing pregnancies with the same sickening predictability.

With so many treatments and subsequent pregnancies, I became very in tune with my own body. One occasion stands out: I was driving to the surgery and feeling very happy because I had a number of positive pregnancy tests to show my doctor. The first of these had revealed an extremely strong line very quickly, and I'd thought: *This one will definitely go to term.*

However, on the drive to the surgery, I felt a sudden sharp pain in my uterus, as if I had been stabbed with a hot poker. The pain went as quickly as it had arrived, but I was left feeling very sick and drained. I knew the pregnancy had been lost.

My doctor tried to reassure me, but I knew. Still, I hoped and prayed desperately that I was wrong. I was aware that the pregnancy hormone would remain in my system for a while, and it was devastating doing a pregnancy test every day and seeing the hormone get weaker and weaker.

I wasn't very far into my pregnancy that time, but it still amazes me how emotionally attached it's possible to become to even the earliest stages of a new life growing inside you, especially when the baby is wanted so much. As far as I was concerned, I hadn't just lost some cells, I had lost my child. It wasn't disappointment that I felt – that's the feeling you get when you burn the dinner that you've just spent hours slaving over, or your local fête is cancelled due to rain. I was crushed.

Each and every time. It made no difference if I was one week pregnant or 14.

I've noticed recently, though, an increasing recognition of how a woman can experience grief at her miscarriage even if it happens before the medical world's general definition of when an embryo becomes a foetus, i.e. at six weeks. I hope this will offer some solace to others going through the same hell that I did. I think this change in attitude is due largely to the rise of social media, where women are able to share their miscarriage experiences easily with others; this, in turn, can spread to traditional media outlets.

The more that miscarriage is talked about, the less of a taboo it will be. When there is no longer a silence around the subject, hopefully women who go on to suffer a miscarriage will have been more prepared for the emotional trauma that cannot be separated from it. They will know that they are likely to feel that their miscarriage is a very lonely grief, and know that they are not alone in this suffering.

Although there seems to be an increased understanding lately of the feelings of women who experience recurrent, early miscarriage, it is by no means a universal compassion. I have found this to be especially prevalent among the general medical profession. To be told constantly that "miscarriages are very common", or "there was obviously something wrong with it", or "I'm sure you'll have better luck next time" soon became almost as hard for me to bear as the miscarriages themselves. Everyone meant well when they said these sorts of things, of course they did. They thought that reassuring me that everything would be all right might help lessen my pain. But there's a very simple reason why this didn't work – I knew there was something wrong with me, not with the poor babies that I had lost. It was *my* body that was to blame. But I just felt so helpless in the face of all the "experts".

During these years of miscarriage, I was also asked by a number of people whether I had thought about adopting. Of course I had. I had considered every possible option to enable me to have the child I longed for, short of stealing one. Mark, though, did not want the responsibility of bringing up another child through adoption. But this didn't make him a bad person. It's important to remember that the only reason he agreed to us having fertility treatment was out of love for me; if I hadn't come along, he would never have thought about having more children.

I've been asked, too, if I think there's any real difference between carrying a donor baby and adopting one. The truthful answer is that I don't know because I've never adopted, but I can imagine very well that the feeling of intense love that adoptive parents feel for their child is as strong as any biological attachment. But to feel my son developing inside me, to give birth to him, knowing that he was safe and well, was the realisation of my dreams. I am William's mother; William is my child – I can't put it any simpler than that.

CHAPTER EIGHT

It's wonderful when the person you have been in a relationship with for a number of years is still able to surprise you, in a nice way of course. In 2005, after six years together, Mark did just that. It was Christmas and we were staying with his parents in Barton, a little village just outside Darlington, North Yorkshire. When we were out shopping with his mother, Judy, in Richmond, which is close by, Mark said he wanted to show me the castle. But it was blowing a gale so neither Judy nor I fancied going.

When we returned to his parents' house, Mark asked me to come outside with him for a minute. It was really cold, so not unsurprisingly I asked why.

"Because it's important," he replied.

Expecting to be shown the garden overrun with Santa's reindeer or something, I stepped outside. No reindeer.

I followed Mark down the path, shivering. He stopped next to the coal bunker and drew me close. Then he put his hand in his pocket and pulled out something small and glittering.

"Will you marry me?" he said.

"What do you mean?" I said.

"What do you think I mean? I want us to get married! Would you like to?"

"Oh, yes, yes, of course!" I felt myself doing that girly, teary-eyed thing.

"Thank God for that."

Mark placed the ring on my finger. It was a beautiful solitaire, something I would have chosen myself. He then explained that he had planned to propose at Richmond Castle. But I was more than happy with the backdrop of a bunker. We hugged and kissed, and I no longer felt the cold.

As we were living in West Swindon at the time, it made sense to get married nearby. So, we booked our wedding at the Swallow Hotel in South Marston, for 29th May, 2005. I ordered my dress from a friend's catalogue, but when a few days before the 29th it still hadn't arrived, I had to buy another one as back-up. It was a good job I did as the original dress evaporated into thin air. The replacement, from Debenhams, was actually a bridesmaid's dress but it didn't look like one. It fitted perfectly too. When I took it to the till, I was told that it was now half-price, so my wedding dress cost me all of £60. It was meant to be.

Because we had a mortgage, childcare expenses and maintenance, school trips, school uniform, music lessons, shoes, clothes, etc. – and fertility treatment to pay for, we had to be careful about our wedding budget. We didn't hire a

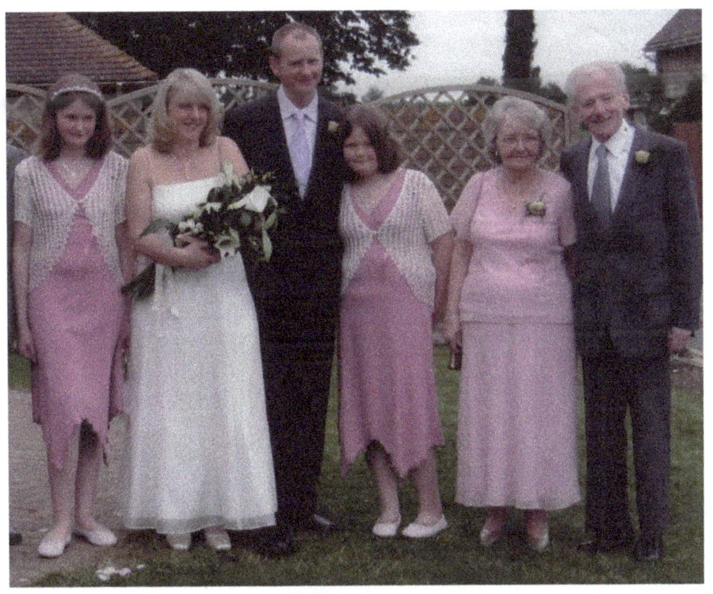

Left to right: May, me, Mark, Evie, Mark's mum and dad

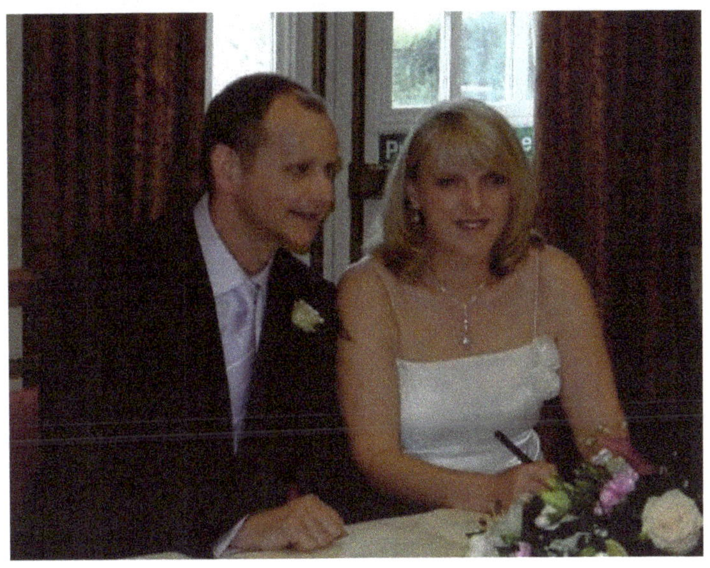

Signing the register

wedding car, and I did my make-up and hair myself, and the hotel's wonderful events manager helped put on my false nails. When I had finished getting ready, she told me to look out of the window. There was a gleaming silver BMW, with wedding bows tied to the bonnet. "Oh, is someone else getting married today as well?" I asked. "No, it belongs to the chef, but he was very happy to lend it to you when I asked," she replied. All the staff at the hotel were great, and made our day so enjoyable, from the wedding breakfast through to the evening reception. It's such a shame that the hotel has since closed down.

A few months later, we went on our honeymoon, to a campsite that we love at Burnham on Sea. It is so beautiful there and we enjoy spending hours walking along the beach. We had booked our pitch in advance but when the weekend arrived it was bucketing down; we decided to go anyway. On arrival, the campsite owner looked at us as if we were mad, and no doubt we looked even madder after battling to put up the tent in the howling wind and rain – we were completely soaked through, despite our waterproofs. We had also just got our first dog together, Jacko, so camping with a noisy, excitable dog in those conditions was a recipe for disaster. Except it turned out to be one of the most enjoyable weekends we've ever had.

Jacko, a beautiful golden Labrador, came into our lives at 11 months old. He belonged to a family from our street but they were planning to give him to a dogs' home. Although they fed him well they were unable to devote the time needed to make him happy, through frequent walks and socialising with other dogs, etc. Before I explain what a wonderful, loving dog Jacko was, I suppose I should say that he did have one character defect – racism! This was particularly noticeable in his behaviour towards a Chinese guy who lived around the corner. Whenever Jacko saw him, he would bark furiously, which frightened the man at first but he soon got used to it. Jacko embarrassed us with this barking, but there was nothing Mark or I could do to stop him.

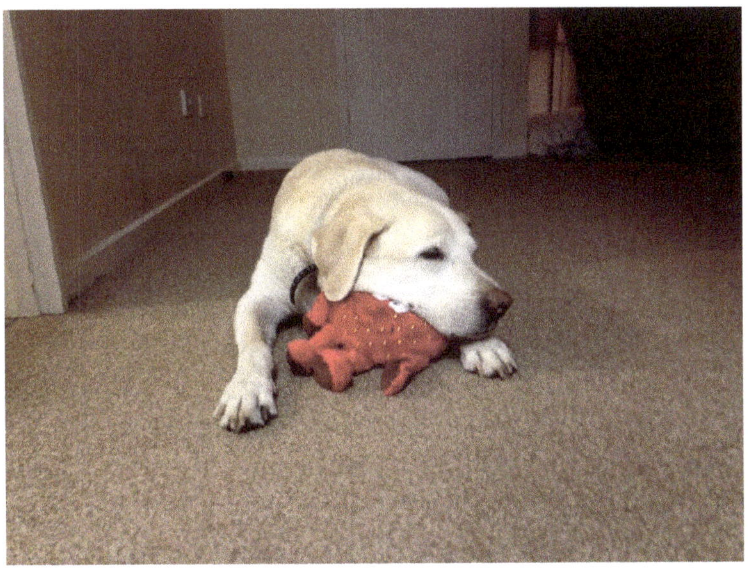

Lovely Jacko

It was shortly after my third miscarriage, at 14 weeks, that we took Jacko into our home. He was with us for over 12 years, and I loved him so much. We tried to give him three walks a day and everywhere we went he came along too. I truly believe that animals have souls – Jacko was so sensitive to my emotions. I'm sure he knew every time I was pregnant as he would never jump up at me then, although he always liked to do this at other times, purely out of affection. Also, whenever I miscarried, he would know this too and would put his head in my lap as I cried. Sometimes I would be unable to stop myself crying for hours, and the whole time he wouldn't move. Jacko was a massive comfort to me, and without him by my side I don't think I would have been able to endure all the years of recurrent miscarriage. In September 2017, we had to have him put down – he was so ill in the end that you could see the pain in his face, despite medication. Having to do this filled me with a grief that was not dissimilar to that I'd felt after my miscarriages. I suppose I had loved him as if he were my child.

CHAPTER NINE

After my last miscarriage, I came terrifyingly close to committing suicide. It was the 6th of May and the baby had survived for about 13 weeks. I was told the news on a Thursday but was unable to have a D&C until the following Monday. I find it almost impossible to describe the all-consuming despair I felt, knowing that the child I was carrying inside me had died.

The night after the D&C, I knew I would never be able to sleep so I just stayed up while Mark went to bed. In fact, my thoughts and emotions were so frantic that I hadn't slept for three nights. It was then that I decided there really was no other way out of my torment but to take away the life I had been given. I felt completely selfish, but my concern for how my family and friends would be affected by my suicide was no longer the preventative measure it had been until then; the combination of crushing exhaustion and sense of utter hopelessness saw to that.

So, I filled a pint glass with water and took all the tablets out of the medicine cabinet and put them on the table. I was determined to put an end to my pain once and for all and began to swallow the tablets. I'm not sure what, in my zombie-like state, made me think of a particular dear friend, but I'm so glad that I did. We had been friends since working together in Germany and are still close today. She lives very near to me, with her son, and was so supportive during these crisis years of loss. Although she is far from narrow minded (I'm not sure we'd be friends if she was), she is very religious. As I was taking the tablets, I remembered one drunken night in Germany when she said, "If you commit suicide you'll go to hell." I'm not sure that the memory of these words alone made me stop what I was doing, after all I would just be swapping one hell for another. I think, rather, that it made me turn my focus to the fact that there must be an alternative to never-ending hell. Although at the time I was far from knowing exactly what this might be, the thought was enough to stop me from continuing with my actions. So, thank you, dear friend, for saving my life, and in doing so giving another new life a chance too.

Other friends were also a great source of solace to me during my miscarriage traumas. Julie Stevenson, a friend from my cabin-crew days, and Lisa Nichols, were always very supportive of me. Samantha Highley was a real shoulder to cry on and would listen to me for hours, such a lovely person and a brilliant friend.

As well as this support, the care given to me by my sister was invaluable. Julie was always there at the end of the phone, and in person whenever possible. I have a great deal of respect and admiration for Julie. After leaving school, she trained to be a chef and worked in this role for a few years. She then decided she wanted a complete change and retrained in business administration, becoming a secretary. After her marriage to David and the birth of their two daughters, she turned to child-minding as a means of earning an income and being able to care for her children at the same time. Once the girls began school, she returned to secretarial work. Then, in her 40s, she made the brave decision to train to be a nurse. For this, she first had to complete a year's Access to HE Diploma (Nursing), followed by a three-year university degree. Although Julie has no regrets about becoming a nurse, she does find working for the NHS incredibly tough, for the same reasons I think most of its workers do.

Julie's husband is a cabinet maker by trade but can turn his hand to pretty much anything practical. Their daughter Catherine, who's now 18, is horse mad, and has a lovely horse of her own called Star. She has just gained a diploma in Equine Studies and we are all very proud of her. Elleka, who's 16, is extremely clever, so much so that a teacher at her state school had contacted Julie to suggest that she would benefit greatly from attending a private school. Encouraged by this, Elleka applied to a public school nearby and passed the entrance test with flying colours. On the back of this, she was offered a scholarship, which she accepted. She loves her school and her current aim is to become either an architect or a space scientist (although I think she could probably manage both at the same time!). She is also a very talented artist. One day, when she was about 12, Julie and I were just chatting together at my house while Elleka was scribbling away with a pencil on a piece of paper. I was stunned when she showed me what she had just quickly produced – an exact replica of the chair in the corner of the room. Perhaps my Grandad Joe had chosen to pass on his artistic genes through Elleka.

In addition to this emotional help from my sister and my friends, I received comfort from a couple of more unexpected sources too. After my last miscarriage, in 2010, I spent hours on the phone to Uncle Bob. He's always willing to listen to me, and his calm nature has the effect of relaxing me too. I also talked to my dad often, and he amazed me with his compassion. But he was still my typical Dad, e.g. frequently telling me that I should go and talk to the vicar about my problems!

Throughout all of those years of repeated pregnancy loss I really did miss my mother. But all these wonderful people helped me through.

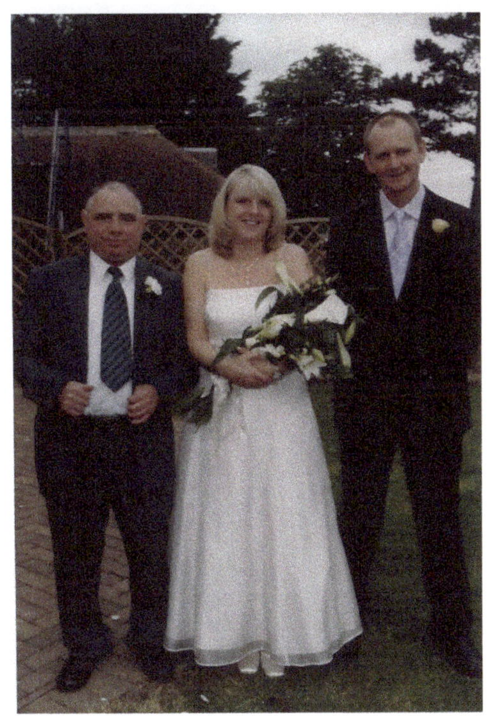

Dad, Me and Mark

CHAPTER TEN

How many miscarriages does it take before medical professionals accept that this must be due to something other than "just bad luck"? Eighteen, it would seem. After years of treatment at St Mary's Hospital in Paddington, still no-one could tell me why I wasn't able to carry a baby to full-term. Even though after my last miscarriage I managed to get the foetus tested in an attempt to establish why it didn't survive, the results were inconclusive, and I don't even know the sex of the baby. In fact, I don't know the sex of any of my lost babies. Sometimes I think this is a blessing, but other times I wonder if it might have helped my grieving process to know and even, perhaps, to have given them a name.

Looking back, it seems shocking that, ultimately, it was left to me to try to find out the reasons for my repeat miscarriages. Even though after the last one I had given up on ever having a child, I knew that I would never be able to rest until the cause of the miscarriages was established. So, it was back to research.

Reading *Is Your Body Baby Friendly?* by Alan E. Beer, M.D. changed everything for me. Because it was this book that led me to Dr Shehata, and it was because of him that I was able, finally, to have a baby of my own. I still have this book, with all the underlining and notes I'd made in the margins, which remind me of the impact the words had on me at the time. Not that I need reminding – the effect of seeing my own exact experiences in print was so powerful it was almost overwhelming. Here was someone telling me that I was not very unlucky, hysterical, or crazy. I was, in fact, right.

This book is not an easy read, on both a technical and emotional level, but this didn't matter at all. I was no longer scared, just determined. I think I would have ploughed my way through a tome on astrophysics if I'd thought it would provide me with the answers I so desperately needed.

Although a number of different causes of infertility and repeat miscarriages are covered comprehensively in *Is Your Body Baby Friendly?*, it was the section dealing with natural killer (NK) cells that I kept coming back to. I was convinced that these cells were the reason why I had not been able to carry a baby to full-term. Now all I needed was to have this confirmed. At the time, I was under the care of Dr Lesley Regan at St Mary's Hospital in London, but her policy was not to test levels of NK cells, so I had to look elsewhere. Further research showed that there were a couple of obstetrician-gynaecologists in the UK at the time who specialised in this area. I chose Dr Hassan Shehata, whose clinic was in London,

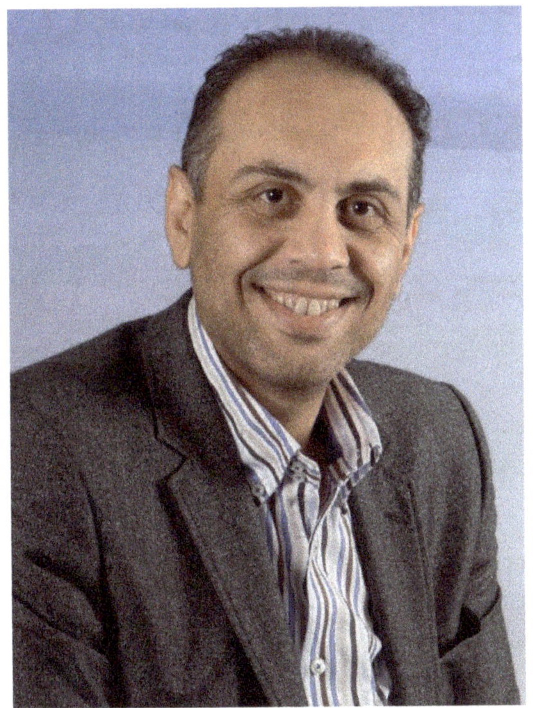

Dr Shehata

and my GP agreed to refer me.

I think it was a few months after my last miscarriage that I first saw Dr Shehata. He was not the slightest bit patronising as I talked about my fertility problems, which was very reassuring after some of my previous experiences. I really felt that he was listening to me, not just to a list of symptoms. I made it clear that I was not looking for treatment, that I could not, mentally, take the risk of another possible miscarriage, so there was not really any financial motive for him to be as caring and patient with me as he was. He understood that I just needed a proper medical explanation as to why I had failed, over and over again, to carry a baby to full-term.

Dr Shehata explained that natural killer cells are a type of white blood cell, and as such are used by the immune system to protect the body against invaders and infectious diseases. So, they are not in themselves something to worry about, but problems can arise when they exist in large numbers and mistakenly see something harmless, in this case a normal embryo/foetus, as a threat to the body. When there are high levels of natural killer cells assuming that the pregnancy is a virus or toxin, they can respond by attacking and killing it.

This is why what had happened to me seemed to make so much sense. With recurrent pregnancy loss, an underlying pathology is usually the cause. Dr Shehata was sure that my own natural killer cells were to blame for my repeated pregnancy loss and implantation failure. He was later proved right in this diagnosis.

This was the light bulb moment I had been searching for. Although the tests carried out by Dr Shehata showed not to be definitive with regard to problems with my own natural killer cells, he was still sure that they were the cause of my infertility.

As I stated in the preface to this story, I hold no claim to medical knowledge regarding recurrent miscarriage and can only say what worked for me. So, it would be remiss of me not to also mention the argument against considering high levels of NK cells to be responsible for failure to carry a baby to full-term. The main focus of this argument is the difference between the NK cells in the blood and those present in the uterus, the latter of which do not appear in circulation but remain in position in the endometrium.

Those experts who do not believe raised levels of blood NK cells can be responsible for early miscarriages obviously do not agree with any treatments offered to reduce these levels. So, before choosing to go down the NK-cells treatment route, it would be wise to discuss it in depth with medical professionals. However, even though investigation into, and treatment of, problems with NK cells in repeat miscarriages is still at the experimental-medicine stage, I firmly believe that it will soon become part of mainstream medicine. In the meantime, for many women who have tried all other options to prevent recurrent miscarriage, without success, treatment focussing on their NK cells is proving to be a triumph.

So, Dr Shehata's advice was encouraging, and I trusted him implicitly, but because I was far too scared at that stage to try for a baby again, I abandoned my dream.

CHAPTER ELEVEN

Although my need for a child of my own had come very close at times to being all-consuming, I can say with confidence that May and Evie never suffered as a result of it, neither emotionally nor financially. I knew right from the start that Mark's daughters were his world and thought it was right that they should always come first. I didn't want their lives to be disturbed any more than they had been already as a result of their parents' divorce. All through my expensive fertility treatment, we always ensured that the girls never went without; it was always Mark and I who bore the brunt, not least through an enforced non-existent social life.

Despite money being very tight when we began our fertility journey, as May and Evie got older our financial situation improved, and once they had reached the age where Mark was no longer required to pay maintenance for their upkeep, things got easier again. But even when Mark was no longer legally obliged to support his children, we both wanted to continue to help them out as much as we could. For example, when May was doing her nursing degree, we used to chip in towards her housing and transport costs, etc., in the hope that she would not be saddled with heavy debts at the start of her adult life.

Not having to spend money on fertility treatment any more meant that Mark and I were now able to spoil ourselves. Meals out, nice clothes, holidays – everything we could now afford to do, we did. I'm not sure if I realised at the time that this was all just a desperate attempt to try to forget about ever having a baby. I threw myself into anything for which motherhood was not a requirement: I was my airline's most enthusiastic cabin-crew member and was promoted to Cabin Supervisor; my little house was the cleanest in Oxfordshire, and Jacko was groomed to perfection. But still. Still, it was there, a magnetic pull that would just not go away.

For four years, I tried. Every time I saw a pregnant woman – and they seemed to be everywhere – I would turn away, but not before helplessly wondering how far they were into their pregnancy, whether it was their first child, whether they were carrying a boy or a girl, whether they were single or had a partner or husband . . . it just went on and on. Whenever family or friends had a new baby, it hurt like hell. To say that I wasn't pleased for them wouldn't be true, but the beautiful weight of the baby in my arms, their pure new breath and the heavenly softness of their skin aroused my longing for a baby of my own to an almost physical level of pain. There were times when this longing was so strong that it terrified me.

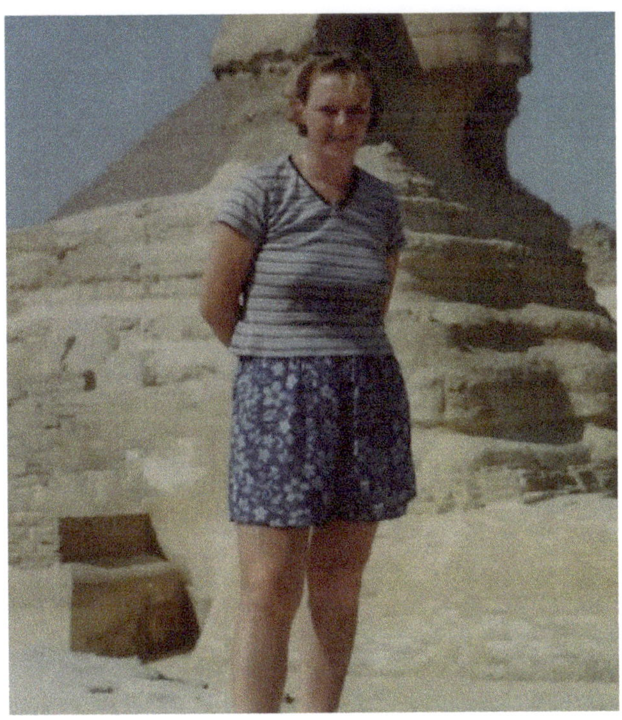

Egypt, with work

Then, tiny whisper by tiny whisper, something was telling me that I should, perhaps, try one more time for a baby. At first, my head shouted down these quiet little murmurings, and I would just agree: "Yes, loud clanging noise in my head, you're quite right; it's hopeless, let's forget it."

But the thought that maybe, just maybe, with the care and expertise of Dr Shehata on my side, I could make it work began to win over the negative internal voice. I decided to confide in my sister – my *nurse* sister, who would know that what I was contemplating was probably, from a medical perspective, just a pipe dream.

We speak regularly on the phone, so Julie wasn't surprised to get my call. After the usual greetings, I came right out with it.

"I want to try one last time for a baby."

Silence.

"Julie?"

More silence.

"Julie – are you still there?"

"Yes, I am."

"I know you must think I'm being ridiculous, at my age –"

"I think it's a great idea."

"– and with all my miscarriages and . . . what did you just say?"

"I said I think it's a great idea."

"You do? Really? Honestly? I mean just say if you think..."

"Look, I know that if you don't at least give it one more try then you'll end up regretting it for the rest of your life."

Julie was right. I knew that not only would I be filled with regret if I didn't follow through on this inescapable wish, I would probably end up embittered and permanently unstable too. Then I could be promoted to Cabin Manager, have my house valued at two million, and Jacko could win Crufts, but it would all mean nothing to me. And I would most probably be such miserable company that Mark would wish he couldn't afford to take me out anywhere.

But, by this time, I was approaching 46, and my age was very much against me. Although the cut-off age for treatment at the Oxford Fertility Clinic using donor embryos was 46, it would have taken a while for any processes to be put in place, so they were unable to treat me, even as a paying client. I then approached a clinic in Cardiff, again as a private client. They also said that they couldn't treat me there, for the same reasons as the clinic in Oxford, but they offered me the option of treatment in a satellite clinic overseas instead – at the cost of £12,000, which we just could not afford.

So, it was back to independent research. I spent days, weeks, on the internet. I searched websites, followed up leads from forums, and contacted anyone I thought might be able to supply me with important information on clinics. I knew the treatment would have to be carried out overseas but was determined that it would be the best possible. I had heard too many horror stories of British people having botched medical treatment abroad, and there was no way I was going to risk the safety of any child I may conceive there. But I had no concerns about the care I would receive in the UK on my return as Dr Shehata would continue my treatment.

After much thought and discussion with Mark, we eventually opted for the Gynem Clinic in Prague, one of the most highly recommended. Their success rate is impressive and the treatment they offer is about half the price of comparable treatment in the UK. The clinic works in conjunction with a company called Medical Travel, which oversees the practicalities, including transport, hotels, pick-ups and drop-offs, etc.

Although during my fertility treatment in the UK the sperm and egg donors had been chosen by the clinic, with the Gynem Clinic we were able to make the choice ourselves. There were no names or photos provided, of course, instead we were given the physical characteristics of each sperm and egg donor to enable us to make our choice. The sperm donor we opted for was tall with blond hair and blue eyes (similar to Mark) and the egg donor had strawberry-blonde hair, greenish-blue eyes and was about 5ft 5 (like me). Dr Shehata prescribed various medications for me to take for four weeks prior to my treatment at the clinic. These included steroids, heparin, aspirin and vitamin E.

As we set off, in February 2015, I was filled with excitement. But there was an element of trepidation involved too – what if the Gynem's glitzy website was covering up an organisation that was actually totally inefficient or, God forbid, just a huge scam? But I needn't have worried; the moment we stepped through the door of the new purpose-built clinic, I knew I was in safe hands. It was exactly as I'd seen in the photos – pristine, full of light and high-tech. But it proved to be more than this; a website can't convey the total professionalism, mixed with genuine empathy, of all the staff. I'm not so naïve as to think that the Gynem exists for entirely philanthropic reasons, but there's no doubting the team really do have their patients' best interests at heart.

The implantation of the donor embryos was a relatively quick process, and I was confident that it stood a fair chance of success; it was the carrying of a baby to full-term that was my problem rather than not getting pregnant in the first place. So, imagine my shock and upset when the treatment that had usually worked for me in the past wasn't successful at the Prague clinic. Flying home, I felt more of a failure than ever before.

But still I didn't give up. I reasoned that using fresh embryos rather than frozen ones might have a greater chance of success and managed to persuade Mark to let us try this instead. We arranged to have this carried out at the same clinic, in June. I knew that this really was my final chance; there was no way Mark would allow me to try again, with any treatment method, anywhere.

Come June, I was due to have a pre-op scan at the clinic, but for some reason I decided to have it in the UK before instead. It was good that I did because the scan showed I had an internal cyst, which meant that the procedure would not have been able to go ahead and I would have had another wasted journey to Prague. But, unfortunately, I had already booked leave from work so began to feel as if everything was going against me all over again. Also, although my periods had always been very regular, this had changed recently and it was becoming increasingly difficult to accurately monitor my cycle. Any fertility drugs have to be taken at exactly the right point in the cycle, so in order to be able to plan the timing of treatment effectively, my periods had to be regular. It was for this reason that I was put on the pill. Taking the contraceptive pill was the suggestion of our Patient Co-ordinator in Prague, Richard Kveck. He was amazing at his job and a wonderful person too.

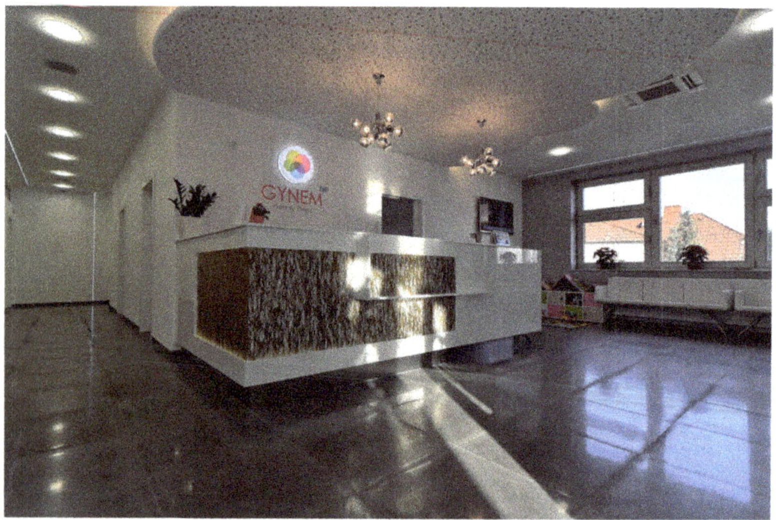

Gynem Clinic

CHAPTER TWELVE

The day after arriving in Prague for the second visit, we were picked up at our hotel by Richard. It was the 30th of September, 2015. I was feeling the usual mixture of fear and excitement but by the time we arrived at the clinic, Richard had managed to calm me down considerably.

The main surgical team consisted of Dr Milan Mrázek and Dr Tomas Rieger. Treatment involved the use of two fresh embryos that were at the blastocyst stage, i.e. that have developed for five days after fertilisation. Dr Rieger carried out the implantation, and the whole process took only about 20 minutes. When the embryos were in position, they appeared on the monitor lit up like tiny stars; it was the most beautiful sight.

After the embryos had been implanted, I had to lie down, with my feet up, for about 30 to 45 minutes. Then it was a taxi ride back to the hotel. On the way, the driver hit the kerb, making me jump, and I was really worried that this might have caused something to go wrong with the treatment.

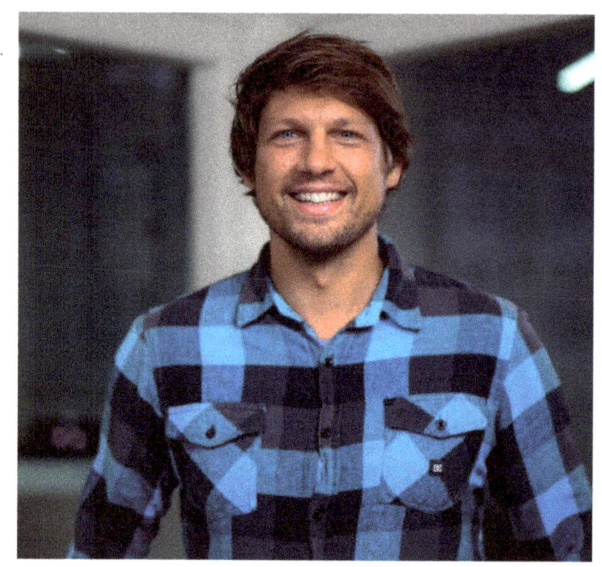

Richard Kveck, Patient Co-ordinator

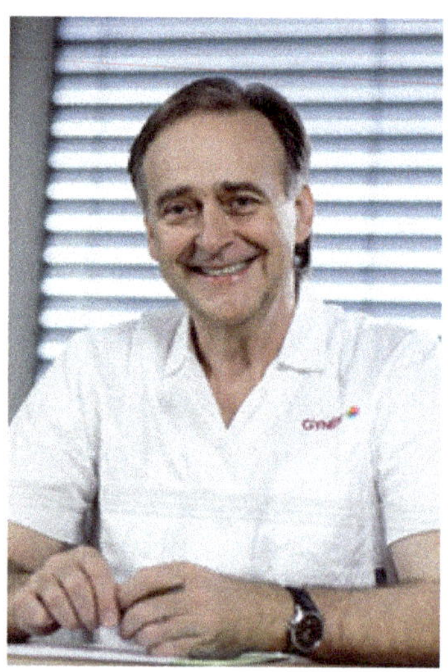

Dr Mrázek

As I talked about earlier, I first took an interest in alternative health therapy when my mum was diagnosed with terminal cancer, and I still believe that it can have huge benefits. Although I didn't stick rigidly to the Gerson Therapy™ during my attempts to carry a baby to full-term, I always ensured that I ate healthily and had the required (large) number of organic fresh juices every day. Just as using this therapy prolonged my mother's life rather than saving it, so the knowledge that I was doing everything I could to give my baby the best chance of survival helped my mental well-being, even though there was no guarantee that it would lead to fulfilment of my dreams.

The Gerson Therapy™ was not the only means of extra support and care that I used to try and get my body to carry a baby to full-term. In support of the IVF medication and the medication prescribed by Dr Shehata to control my natural killer cells, I took vitamin E supplements daily to strengthen my defence against illness, and salmon oil for its Omega 3 fatty acids, which regulate reproductive hormones and increase blood flow to the uterus, helping the uterine lining to develop. I also took Siberian ginseng capsules to reinforce my body's chi, or vital energy, and maca root, a superfood that aids the pituitary, adrenal and thyroid glands, which are involved in aiding hormonal balance. As well as taking these important supplements, I followed the Fertility Diet both when I was trying to get pregnant and during pregnancy. I used alternative therapy to help my mental well-being too: meditation for relaxation, and visualisation, e.g. imagining holding my baby and feeding and looking after him. In addition, I had acupuncture regularly with Ke Wang, in Witney, which helped me enormously to maintain positivity.

I knew by now that all these alternative therapies alone weren't going to ensure that my baby would survive through gestation, but I also knew that to not do them would be, in some way, an admission of defeat. So, I adhered to the juicing regime. Because the juice had to be freshly prepared, on our first visit to Prague we had to go across town three times a day for it. But by the time of our second visit, a new juice bar had opened very close to the hotel and Mark was able to just pop over and collect the juice for me; I took this as a positive sign from above.

As it turned out, I didn't leave the hotel room for five days! I wanted to ensure the embryos had implanted properly before flying home, just in case there was any risk attached to being at high altitude.

We flew back on the sixth day. I managed to wait only two more days before doing a pregnancy test, using a kit from Boots that is able to give a result four days earlier than standard kits. Although the line that showed was very faint, it was there.

I think this would be a good place to mention my extreme impatience when it came to testing for most of my pregnancies, and how this, on occasions, led to disappointment that could have been avoided if I had been willing to wait a little longer. By this I mean that I might never have known about the eight 'chemical pregnancies' if I hadn't been so desperate to find out the results, and I could probably have saved myself a lot of heartache. This is especially true given my strong beliefs about the early stage at which life starts. I knew that it was unwise to carry out pregnancy tests before the recommended time had elapsed after possible conception, but I just could not stop myself.

I realise that some people might think my 'obsession' with having a baby of my own was in some ways selfish, and that constantly checking if I was pregnant before it was medically advisable to do so only added to the pressure that Mark was under with the whole process. I can understand this. But all I can do is repeat that my longing for motherhood was so strong that it always overcame all rational thought, making me as helpless as a mouse before a lion.

It would not surprise me either if some worry that my son, as he grows older and begins to understand the background to his birth, might also feel under pressure. To be the whole world to another person in a huge responsibility. What if William grows up thinking that in order to truly fulfil his mother's dream he has to be perfect? What if he feels he has to stay close to his mother when other children would be ready to flee the nest? These are things that concern me too. But I will do my utmost to make sure that William knows I have no expectations of him other than to always be kind and honest. I want him to choose how he lives the life that I have given him.

CHAPTER THIRTEEN

So, my pregnancy test was positive, but rather than take any chances, I did nothing during the remainder of my leave, apart from a bit of light housework. Then I pulled a big sickie from work. I told them I was suffering from high blood pressure and couldn't fly, which was true, but I omitted to mention the fact that I was also pregnant. It wasn't until I was seven weeks' pregnant that I told my supervisor but asked her not to tell anyone else. Then, at nine weeks, I told my manager but again asked her to please keep the information to herself for the time being.

I had taken responsibility for ensuring there was continuity in the treatment I was receiving from Dr Shehata and the Gynem Clinic; there was no direct liaison between them.

Dr Shehata had arranged for me to see him at seven, nine and 11 weeks. It was the first scan, at seven weeks, that showed just one of the implanted embryos had been successful. It was also at this time that Dr Shehata told me that once the heartbeat is discernible, the chance of losing the baby is less than 1%. I replied that if this was the case then I must have been very, very unlucky in the past.

How I would have loved to have been able to relax and enjoy this pregnancy, but I was terrified the whole way through. I was so worried about miscarrying again that I did a pregnancy test almost every day for the first three months. The line was getting stronger and stronger but I knew that if it began to get lighter I had probably lost my baby. At about nine weeks' gestation, I saw that I had leaked some blood. It was the tiniest amount, no more than a pin prick really, but this was exactly what had happened before my last miscarriage. I was in a complete panic, so distraught that I was unable to drive myself to hospital and one of Mark's colleagues (a lovely man called Butch) kindly gave me a lift. They did a scan, and I was shocked but obviously so relieved too when they said that the baby was fine.

Because Dr Shehata was concerned about me having to travel such a long distance to see him, he referred me back to the John Radcliffe Hospital after the 11-week scan. So, it was back to hospital in Oxford for my scan at 12 weeks. I was so agitated in the waiting room that I kept pacing around and couldn't sit down even when Mark told me that I must. Oh, the relief when I was told there were no problems with that scan either.

But this relief didn't last. I began to worry again almost immediately and imagined that even the most harmless-seeming thing was a sign that something was wrong with my baby. For example, during all my other pregnancies, I couldn't stand the smell of coffee – it made me feel really sick – but this time I had no problem with it at all. That must mean that I wasn't pregnant anymore. Paranoid thoughts like this rarely left me.

Even though at the start of the treatment at the Gynem Clinic I made myself view it as just a clinical experiment, to try to protect my mental health, I couldn't keep this up for long and soon became extremely attached to the baby growing inside me. I suppose this was inevitable really. However, I did have counselling once a week throughout the pregnancy to help support my mental well-being.

At 13 weeks, I woke up one morning unable to breathe properly. I went straight to my GP who, concerned that I may have suffered an embolism, arranged for me to be admitted to hospital. Here, they said I had to have an X-ray, which I was very much against because I didn't want to risk any harm to my baby. But I was forced into having one anyway and, thankfully, it showed no sign of an embolism. My breathing difficulties were put down to a panic attack.

I went back to work in January, on ground duty, but I was still frightened to tell everyone I was pregnant in case I jinxed things. This wasn't rational, of course, but rational was the very last thing I was then. I'm pretty sure that most people at work, well, the women at least, had guessed that I was pregnant anyway – I was big almost from the start. When I was only 13 weeks' pregnant and visiting my dad, one of his friends (who didn't know I was expecting) had said to me, "Cor, Louise, you've put weight on, haven't you?"! It was only when my 16-week scan showed all was well that I felt confident enough to tell my colleagues my news. They were so happy for me.

Shortly after having the X-ray to check for an embolism, I began to develop horrific migraine-like headaches that were so painful they made my eyes water. Because I was pregnant and because of my history of miscarriages, my GP arranged for me to see a neurologist. Dr Buckley, the neurologist, was lovely, and after a thorough examination said she didn't think it was necessary to carry out a brain scan, but she would get a second opinion from a fellow consultant. So, I went home but, in the afternoon, received a phone call from Dr Buckley saying that it had been decided that I should have a brain scan after all.

The results shocked me: I had had a number of Transient Ischaemic Attacks (TIAs), which are a bit like mini strokes. This information made me think that the breathing problems I had at 13 weeks probably had nothing to do with anxiety but were the result of a TIA.

It wasn't possible to have further investigative tests done on the TIAs until after William was born. Then, the first step was to have an MRI scan, and this was followed by a cerebral angiogram. The latter involves the use of a dye, which is carried to the brain via an insertion in the groin. When the dye reached my brain, it felt very strange, as if fireworks were going off in my head. Finally, in March 2018, I was diagnosed with Moyamoya syndrome (which differs from Moyamoya disease in that it occurs in association with other risk factors or conditions). According to the website 'rarediseases.info. nih.gov':

"Moyamoya disease is a rare, progressive, blood vessel disease caused by blocked arteries at the base of the brain in an area called the basal ganglia. The name 'moyamoya' means 'puff of smoke' in Japanese and describes the look of the tangled vessels that form to compensate for the blockage. Affected people are at increased risk of blood clots, strokes, and transient ischemic attacks (TIAs) which are frequently accompanied by seizures and muscular weakness, or paralysis on one side of the body. Affected people may also have disturbed consciousness, speech deficits (usually aphasia), sensory and cognitive impairments, involuntary movements, and vision problems."

In an odd way, this diagnosis was reassuring because it provided an explanation for memory loss that had been bothering me for some time. It also made me wonder whether Moyamoya had been connected to my miscarriages, although my neurologist ruled this out. But, mostly, the diagnosis added to my worries for William's future under my care. I asked the consultant for a prognosis but he said it was not possible to say for sure: "You could have another 30 years, or it could be lights out as soon as you leave my office." Great.

I try to tell myself that nobody knows how long they will have on this earth, but it does little to make me feel better.

Living with Moyamoya feels like having a time bomb inside my head and never knowing when it's going to explode. Yes, I could have another 20–30 years, or I could be rendered permanently disabled from a severe stroke or fall down dead tomorrow. All I want is to be able to nurture William to the best of my ability, into adulthood, and know that he has a good and happy life.

CHAPTER FOURTEEN

The next 16 weeks passed with me in a state of more or less constant agitation, just willing the time to pass. The first thing I had asked my midwife was at what stage a baby could be born safely and she'd replied that for a baby born at 28 weeks the chance of survival was quite high. To try and calm my anxiety, a friend gave me a hand-held Doppler foetal monitor so that I could have the reassurance of hearing the baby's heartbeat whenever I needed to. My midwife advised against this, and I can understand why, but I soon got addicted to it. Also, every night, I would lie still and hope to feel kicking, but because the placenta was at the front (anterior placenta), it took ages for me to feel anything; the first kick I felt wasn't until Easter, after I had just eaten some chocolate.

At 32 weeks, I was told there was something wrong with the placenta and I was admitted to hospital. The placenta was still functioning sufficiently to keep my baby alive but not to support any more growth. This sent me into absolute hysteria, a complete meltdown. Mark wasn't with me because he was in Yorkshire visiting his father, who was suffering from cancer. After three days, the staff told me that it was safe for me to go home but I refused and kept screaming at them, "Get my baby out now!". I was in such a state that they decided to ask a hospital psychiatrist to talk to me. He didn't know my medical history so I had to tell him (okay, I shouted) about all my miscarriages. I genuinely believed that if I were to leave the hospital I would lose this baby.

It took a long time for the psychiatrist's reasoning to sink in and calm me down. Although I was still very unhappy, I eventually agreed to go home, on the proviso that I would have the baby delivered at 37 weeks, instead of the planned 39, and I would have a Doppler scan at the hospital every Monday, Wednesday and Thursday until then.

Around this 32-week stage, a friend at work said that she would like to have a baby shower for me, but I was adamant that I didn't want one. Again, it was the stupid fear of jinxing the safe delivery of my baby. But her request did make me realise that I really had to start buying at least the basics for a new baby – I had nothing, not even a Babygro. So, we bought a pram – wow!

Two weeks before William's new due date, I was waiting outside the John Radcliffe for a lift back home after a Doppler scan when I got a call from the hospital on my mobile. They were not happy with my blood pressure and the Doppler scan and had decided I should be readmitted. So, I went back inside, where I remained for another three days.

The pressure of Mark's father's illness had a devastating effect on Mark's mother. Les and Judy had been together since they were 15 and loved each other deeply. She had been visiting him in hospital for weeks, as had Mark on his days off. When Les was told that his cancer was terminal, the upset to Judy was so great that she suffered a heart attack and ended up in hospital herself. On the 21st of May, Mark was driving back home after visiting his parents when I got a phone call from the hospital in Darlington, asking to speak to Mr Warneford. I explained the situation, but they refused to tell me what was wrong, obviously following hospital procedure. As Mark didn't have a hands-free phone, he never answered calls while driving. So, in order for him to realise that I needed to speak to him urgently, I phoned him repeatedly, without leaving a message. When he did pull over and phoned me back, I told him about the call from the hospital. Although he was very close to home then, he turned around and drove all the way back to Darlington.

But, as I had guessed, and I think Mark had too, his mum had already died. The whole family was shattered. Mark was an only child and so close to his parents. Judy was a lovely woman, even though she always spoke her mind. We all miss her a lot. May and Evie adored her and she felt the same way about them. The girls used to love to go and stay with their grandparents in Barton, and Judy always spent time and effort on choosing gifts that were just right and special for each one.

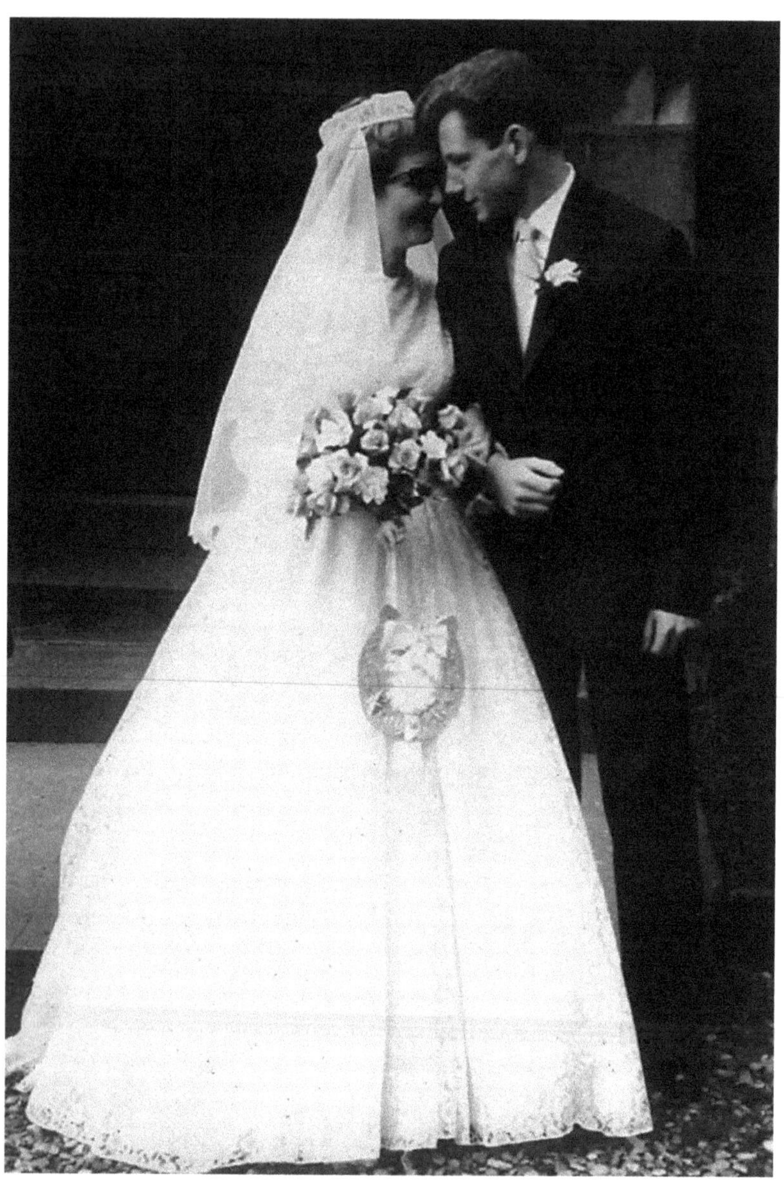

Mark's parents' wedding day

Poor Mark, his head must have been exploding with anguish at this time. But he continued to support his family as he has always done, calmly and lovingly. Even after all these years, I still think he's amazing, and I will always be so thankful that he chose me as his partner in life. Understandably, he needed to stay in Barton with his dad for a while, so I had to face the placenta problem mostly on my own.

As William was originally due to be delivered on June 22nd, I worked up until 10th May. Bringing forward the delivery date to 1st June meant I didn't have as much time to prepare myself mentally as I'd first thought. Not that it would have made much difference as I wasn't able to relax anyway, regardless of how much I tried.

Because of all my health problems, it was decided that the safest thing for both me and the baby would be to admit me to hospital a week before the caesarean. Unsurprisingly, I was the oldest pregnant woman there at the time. The staff were wonderful, so kind to me and interested in the build-up to where I was now.

CHAPTER FIFTEEN

May 31st – I couldn't sleep that night from excitement. I put my hands on my stomach and said, "I'm going to meet you tomorrow!"

By morning, my feeling of anticipation was going through the roof. The caesarean was scheduled for 8.30 am, and Mark and I were told to go down to a little pre-op room until we were called. We waited. And waited. And then waited some more. We were told that the delay was being caused by some emergency admissions, so we understood perfectly, but the tension was still excruciating. We waited so long that when I was eventually called I would have run to the operating theatre if I hadn't been so huge.

I was given an epidural so experienced no pain, just an unpleasant, odd feeling when the needle was inserted. Although I was fully conscious throughout the operation, it still felt as if I was dreaming. Surely this couldn't be me, about to hold my own baby in my arms for the first time?

At 14.07, our little boy was born, weighing 4lbs 15oz.

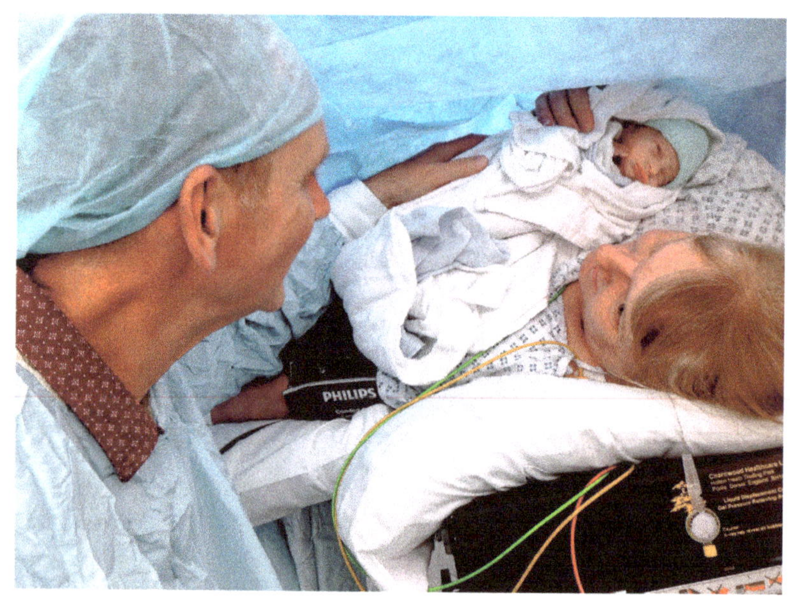

Shortly after William's birth

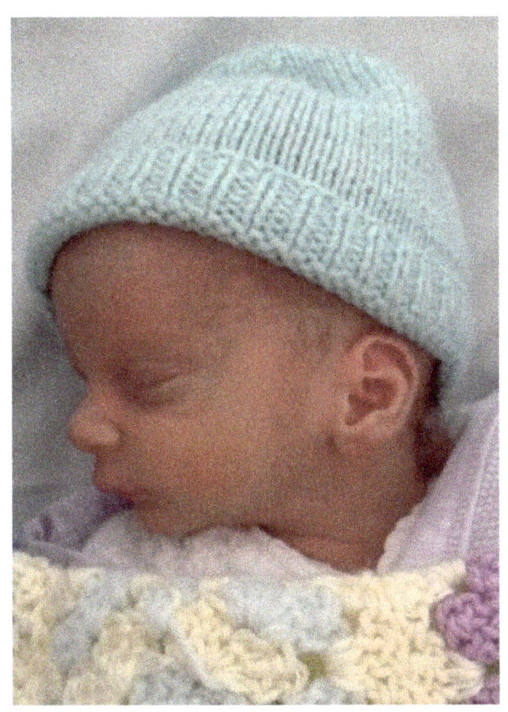

William

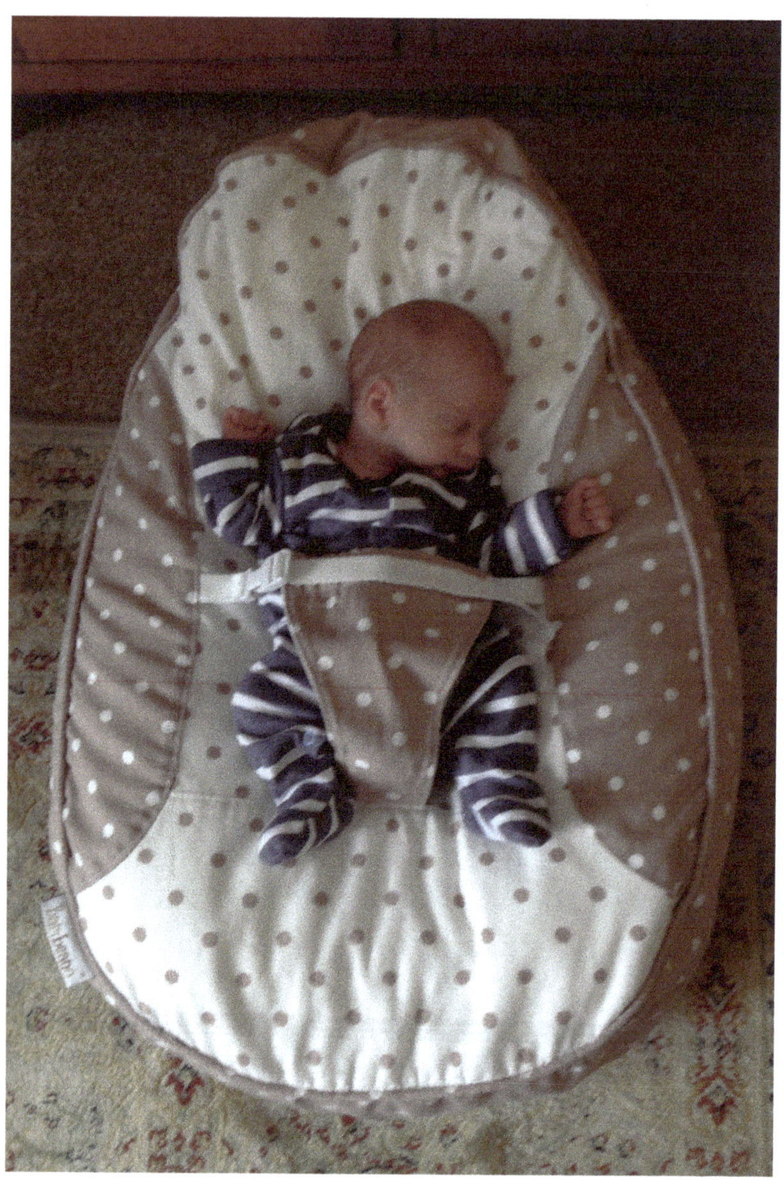

William when he was tiny

He didn't cry for a few seconds after delivery, but to me it felt like minutes, so it was such a relief when he did start to bawl. As soon as he was delivered, he was checked over to make sure he was okay, and he passed all the tests. Our baby was fine. We had chosen not to be told the baby's sex and I was so happy that Mark now had a son.

William's relatively low birth weight did surprise me and, to be honest, worried me a bit too. I couldn't understand how he could be so small when his host body had been so large – I had put on over four-and-a-half stone during the pregnancy. But the midwives assured me that there was no problem with William's weight and that no special care was needed for him.

The next day, Mark had to return to Yorkshire, to help look after his father and arrange his mother's funeral. I remember standing looking out of the ward window, with William in my arms. I watched Mark let Jacko out of the car to have a wee before driving off. To see the man I loved, William's father, have to go away like that made me feel so sad, for all three of us.

I couldn't take my eyes off my wonderful gift from above. Really. I didn't sleep for a couple more nights after his birth. Eventually, the midwife took him away from me, forcing me to get some shut-eye. If it hadn't been for the visitors I received during the daytime, all wanting to cuddle this precious new boy, I think I may well have never put him down. My sister came to visit two days after the birth and was over the moon that she was an aunty at last. May and Evie also came to see their little brother and were delighted with him. It also meant

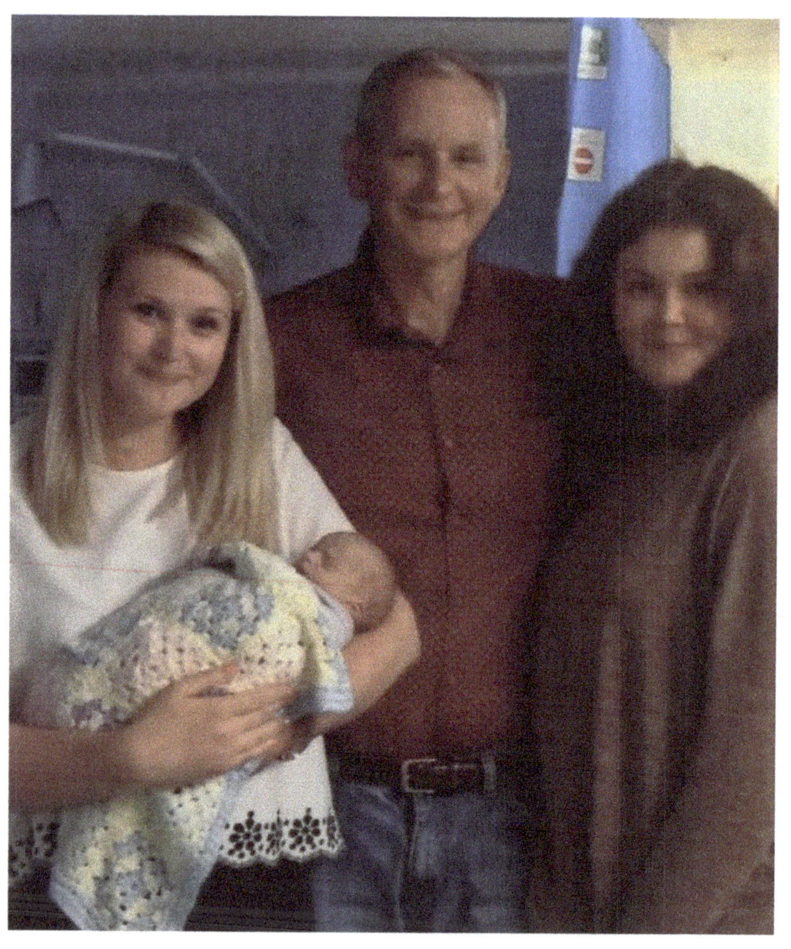

May (holding William), Mark and Evie

a lot to me when two of my friends, Clair and Lisa, came to see us. Lisa and I used to go running and dog-walking together and we had many conversations about my fertility issues.

I stayed in hospital for ten days after William was born because there was no one at home to give me the help that's required after a caesarean and also because I had suffered pre-eclampsia, which still required monitoring. I made use of this time to attend some basic baby-care classes being run by the midwives. We were shown how to bath babies properly and change their nappies, etc. – simple things, but I needed all the reassurance I could get that I was doing things properly. I still worried though. This anxiety soon made its way into my dreams. I had nightmares that someone had stolen my tiny new baby and dropped him out of the window next to my bed.

CHAPTER SIXTEEN

When the day came to take William home, I first got one of the midwives to check that he was okay in the baby car seat. With her assurance, we set off, Mark driving his son for the very first time.

Because I still had most of my pre-baby weight, the seatbelt was tight, and the caesarean site was tender, but I didn't care.

"This is just incredible, isn't it?" I said. "After everything we've been through, we've finally got a baby of our own. I'm so happy!"

"Me too!" Mark beamed and gently patted my leg. "I love you both so much."

I looked round at William, then at his Dad, and gave a sigh of contentment. "And I love you both too, more than I could ever say."

So many times I had imagined pulling up in our driveway, bringing a new baby home. And now it was actually happening.

After letting ourselves in, we put William on the floor, still in his car-seat. It was time to introduce him to Jacko.

Even though I knew how good natured Jacko was, I still felt a bit nervous in case he didn't take to this strange new arrival on his territory. But I needn't have worried; he just hobbled over to William, sniffed him and then lay down next to him. He rarely deviated from this protective position for the remainder of his life. A couple of days after our return home, the health visitor called around, but Jacko wouldn't let her near William at first. I'm sure he sensed that I had finally achieved my dream, and he wasn't going to let anyone take it away from me.

Having to leave the professional expertise and care of the hospital wasn't easy. The worry that something might happen to my baby that I wouldn't know how to deal with remained at the forefront of my mind. At one point, I was convinced William couldn't breathe because he kept on snuffling, and it was only when both my sister and May said this was probably just mucous remaining from his caesarean birth that I relaxed. A bit.

I had not liked the wait involved before breast-feeding after having a caesarean and neither had I liked the excruciating pain involved when I did attempt it, nor William's refusal to drink. It seemed to me that my baby was just not getting any nutrition at all, so I decided to bottle-feed him. Because of his low birth weight, he had to be fed every two hours for the first six weeks and every three hours after that. Right from the start, Mark has always done his share of looking after William and this included the bottle-feeding. We had to set an alarm

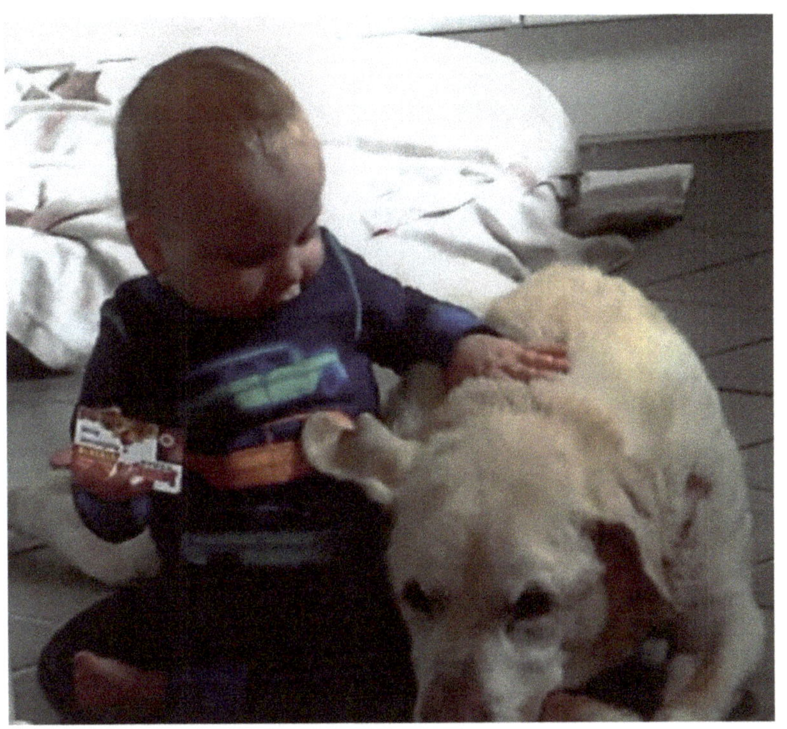

William and Jacko loving each other

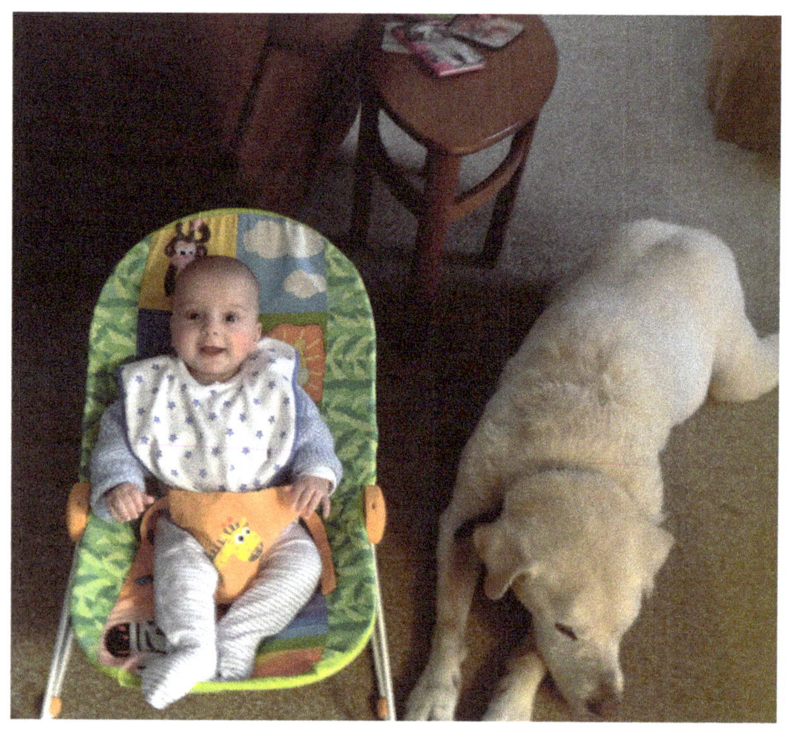

William and Jacko

to enable us to stick to the schedule. Both Mark and I are fortunate to not be too adversely affected by lack of sleep, a result of all the night flights and time-zone changes involved in our jobs, so we were mostly fine with what would probably be exhausting for others. After 22 years working as a flight steward, I wasn't going to be defeated by a few months of tiredness.

Mark had had to use some of his two weeks' paternity leave to help his dad, so I was on my own with William on occasions. But I was lucky to have lots of visitors – family and friends were keen to meet our little miracle, and we had so many gifts and cards. Everyone was overjoyed for us.

Our first outing with our new son consisted of a visit to M&S in Witney to buy some pre-term baby clothes, necessary because of William's unexpectedly low birth weight. This shopping trip was memorable for also being the first, but by no means the last, time that Mark and I were mistaken for grandparents. A very posh elderly lady, wearing a long, colourful scarf leaned over the pram and said, "What a beautiful grandchild you have." When I replied that he was, in fact, our own baby she just said, "Wonderful!" I really don't mind if people make this assumption when they see us with William; it's perfectly understandable.

CHAPTER SEVENTEEN

Once Mark had returned to his job, working consecutive shifts, we usually spent his days off in Yorkshire. This was a stressful time for both of us, with all the travelling and seeing to both William's needs and those of Mark's dad. But it wasn't to be for very long because his dad died a few months later. We're sure that he didn't want to live after Judy had gone. He refused to have a carer even though we offered to pay for one. A friend of his and Judy's, Val, used to go around often to check he was okay, but she couldn't be expected to be there all the time. There were occasions we visited when he just lay in his bed, almost unconscious. When he had returned from a stay in hospital, a nurse had come around every day to give him an insulin injection, but after six weeks he was expected to do the injecting himself. But, of course, he didn't. This is something a carer could have done for him, but we couldn't force him into accepting help.

The day Mark's dad died, Mark had been trying to get

hold of him to say that we wouldn't be able to make it up to Yorkshire as planned because William had a bad cold and we didn't want to risk passing it on. Mark kept ringing all day but there was no answer, so at 8pm he phoned one of his dad's friends to ask if he would pop over and see if he was alright. After having to climb through a window, his friend found that Mark's dad had died in his bed. It was 27th September and he was 77. For the short time that he was with William, he got very attached to him, and I'm sure that Judy would have adored her grandson too.

I can't really comprehend how Mark managed to cope with the tragedy of losing both parents, so close together, especially when he had such a strong, loving bond with them. When my mother passed away, I know that I wanted to go with her to make sure she arrived in the next world safely. I felt this in some ways after my miscarriages, too, and choose to believe that Mum is looking after these lost babies now.

Because of us having to go to Yorkshire to help with Mark's father, my dad didn't get to meet William until he was a couple of months old. He was thrilled by his new grandchild as well as relieved for me. Although William doesn't see him as often as I would like – his house is not child friendly and his ill health makes it impossible for him to travel far – they still have a strong bond.

So, these trips to Yorkshire in the first few months after William's birth made it even more difficult for me to just relax and enjoy my new baby. Of course, this was no-one's fault,

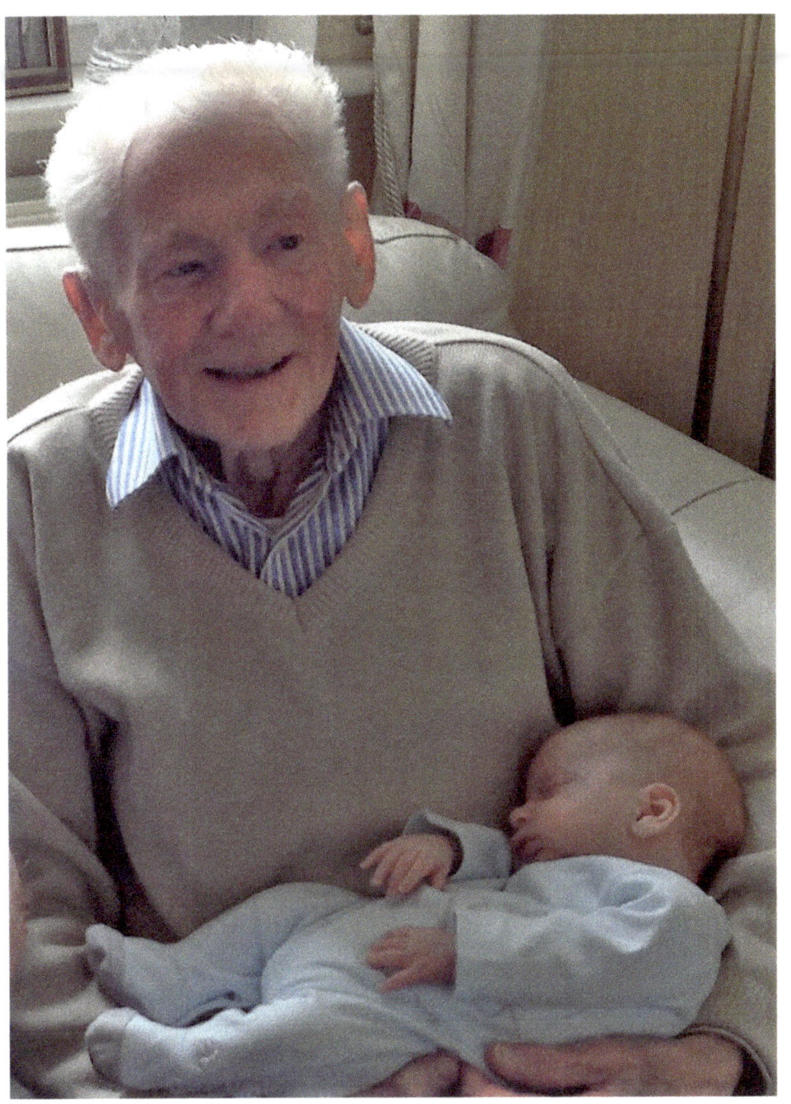

Mark's dad with William

and I certainly don't regret the time we spent with Mark's dad towards the end, but it took its toll. My nightmares where some harm befell William continued. When he was a few weeks' old, I asked the health visitor at what age the danger of Sudden Infant Death Syndrome usually passes, and she replied that it was after about ten months. When May told me about an alarm device that can be attached to a nappy to monitor the rise and fall of the baby's stomach, I bought one straightaway and then used it whenever William was sleeping, day or night, for at least a year. I only stopped when my sister said to me, "Soon he's going to pull that thing off and throw it at you!"

My physical health after William's birth also made things more difficult. Julie, my friend who had been so supportive during the years of trying for a baby, once again stepped to the fore. I had De Quervain's Tenosynovitis and Carpal Tunnel Syndrome in both wrists, which started during the pregnancy, and she babysat on two occasions when I had to go to hospital for day surgery.

Okay, confession time: When William was a couple of months old, I started smoking again. I still can't believe I did this. My greatest wish had finally come true, but I couldn't cope with it. Couldn't cope with my beautiful baby boy. I don't mean the practicalities; it was the enormity of everything I had gone through to achieve this dream that seemed to press in on me from all sides. How could someone so emotionally scarred possibly be trusted to bring up a child? My head was

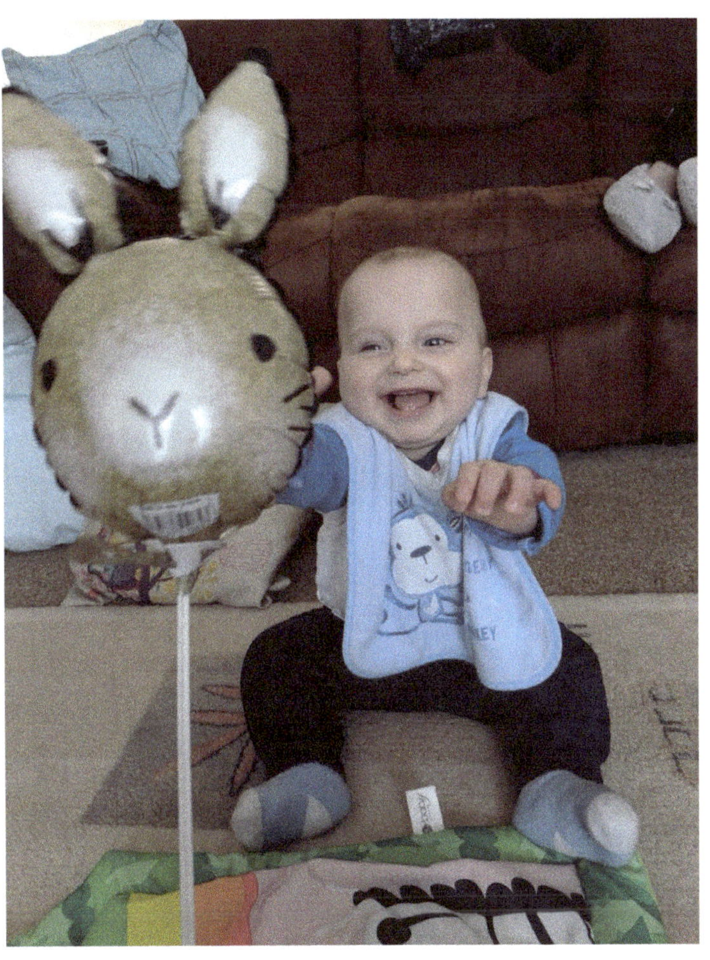

as messed up as my post-baby body. Some mothers turn to alcohol or drugs; I just turned to smoking. Mark smoked and there was plenty of tobacco and Rizlas in the house. I'd been smoking for a number of years but always stopped months before my fertility treatment.

Although Mark and I never smoked around William, it was obvious that he would still suffer from our habit because of how unfit it made us. If we wanted to be around to see our son grow into adulthood, we knew it was important to keep as fit and strong as possible. So, giving up smoking permanently seemed the only option. Once again, Mark was by my side in this, agreeing to give up smoking too. We were helped greatly by a book called *The Easy Way to Stop Smoking*, by Allen Carr, and followed this by attending a motivational talk at the Allen Carr Clinic in London. And it worked – neither of us has smoked since.

CHAPTER EIGHTEEN

Although there is no doubt that my experiences have had a permanent effect on me, I think I have retained the same core elements of my personality that I had as a child: reliability (I hate letting people down), kindness and consideration for others. I can also be a bit ditsy at times (I blame my mother). One of the character traits most important to me, though, is honesty, and a friend once said, "I can't believe how honest you are". I dislike liars very much, and before I allow someone new into my life (particularly after the bad experience with my first few boyfriends), I have to know that I can trust them totally. Mark is equally as honest as I am, so I really hope that with us as role models William will grow up to have absolute integrity too.

I would be so pleased if William develops a love for walking as a pastime, like his parents. But I wouldn't be quite so pleased if he develops a love for motorbikes, like his father. When Mark and I had just bought our first house together, we'd spent all our savings on the deposit and had no money left for furniture,

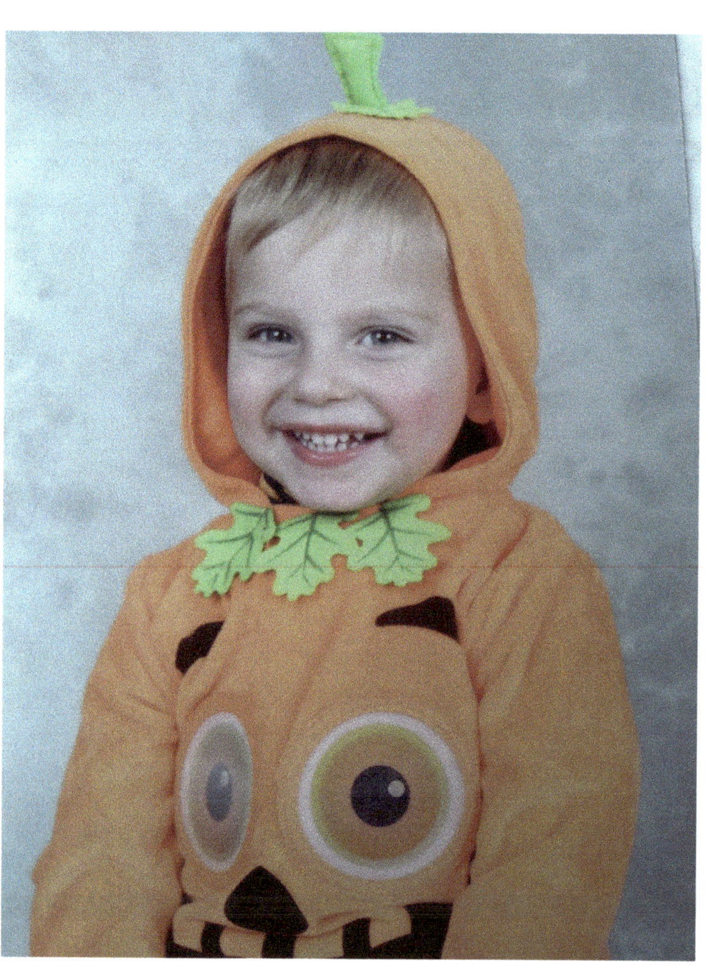

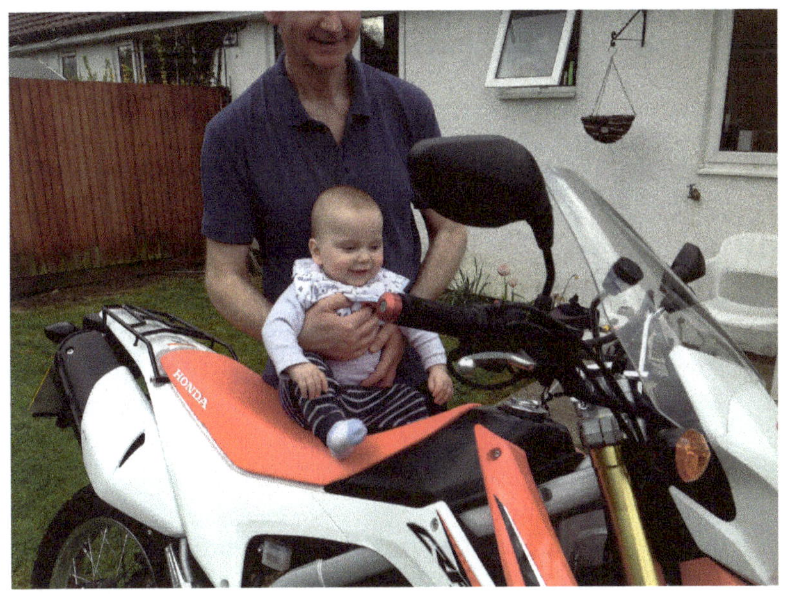

Nice try, Mark

etc., and I had to do the cooking on a portable two-plate hob. One day I was frying some eggs when I heard a motorbike pull up outside. I guessed it would be Mark as he often took bikes out for a trial spin, so I just ignored it. Then Mark popped his head around the door and said, "Hey, Louise, come and see this!" So, I went out, just to humour him, and saw a big, shiny motorbike parked in the drive. "Yes, very nice," I said, and then went to go back inside. "I'm glad you like it," he said, "because I've just bought it." I can't remember exactly what I shouted in response but it definitely contained swear words. I then charged back into the kitchen, picked up the frying pan, stormed back outside and threw it at Mark's (helmeted) head! Do I ever feel guilty about this? Nope.

I would be surprised if William grew to share some of our other likes and hobbies, due to the generation gap if nothing else. For example, as far as music is concerned, in addition to Bruce Springsteen, I enjoy listening to an assortment of different music including rock. I particularly like Bryan Adams (I went to a couple of his concerts when I was living in Germany), André Rieu, The Script and The Verve. Also, William's favourite radio and TV shows (if such things still exist when he reaches adulthood) are likely to be different from mine: I like Jeremy Vine on both TV and radio, films, documentaries – in particular *Britain's Best Walks with Julia Bradbury* – property programmes and detective/police procedural dramas. I very rarely watch any soaps as I find them too stressful and depressing.

My idea of an enjoyable night out has changed over the years, which is no doubt a natural part of growing older, but it also has something to do with the fact that since having William I have less time and energy. These days, I'll settle for a nice meal, or a trip to the cinema, with Mark. Since William's birth, we've actually only been out in the evenings twice, and that was to a 60th birthday party and a retirement do. But after my most cherished dream has finally come true, I'm certainly not about to complain about the increasingly saggy social life that accompanies it. Julie, my friend, babysat on the first occasion and May on the next. May currently lives in Wootton Bassett with her partner Bill and although she doesn't have a child herself, I trust her implicitly to look after her brother. The fact that she's a Health Visitor also comes in handy whenever I'm unsure or worried about some aspect of William's development, etc. How lucky I am to have both a sister and a stepdaughter with nursing degrees! Although Evie, who lives in Tadpole Garden Village in Swindon with her husband Ryan, also adores her brother, it would not be easy for her to babysit as she has a little one of her own, Nancy, to look after. So Nancy is our precious little granddaughter and William's niece. Evie works hard two or three days a week while her mother and Ryan's mother take it in turns to have Nancy, and we help whenever we can.

I have had great affection for May and Evie since the

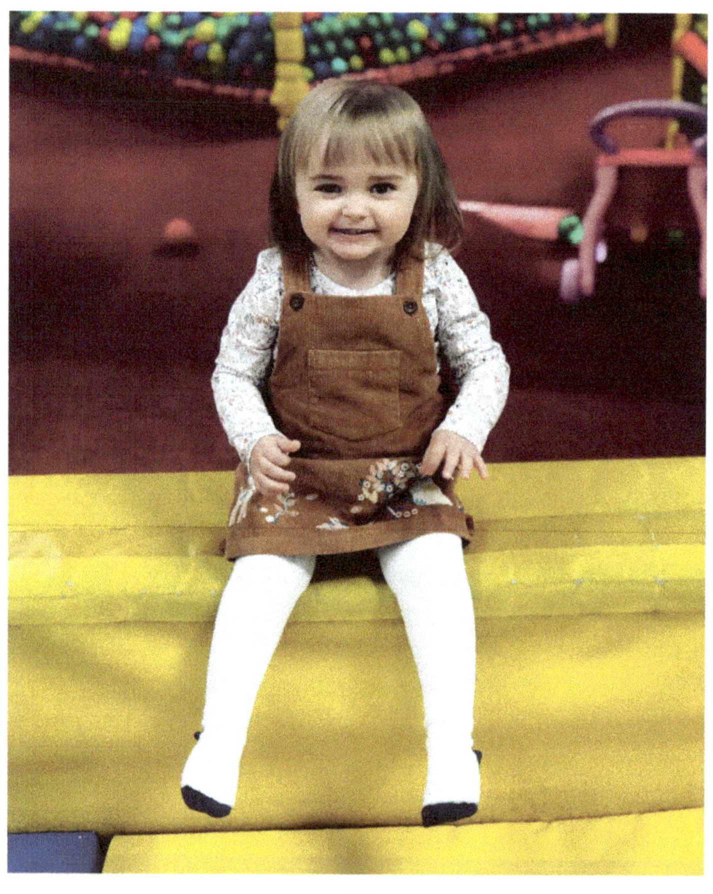

Nancy

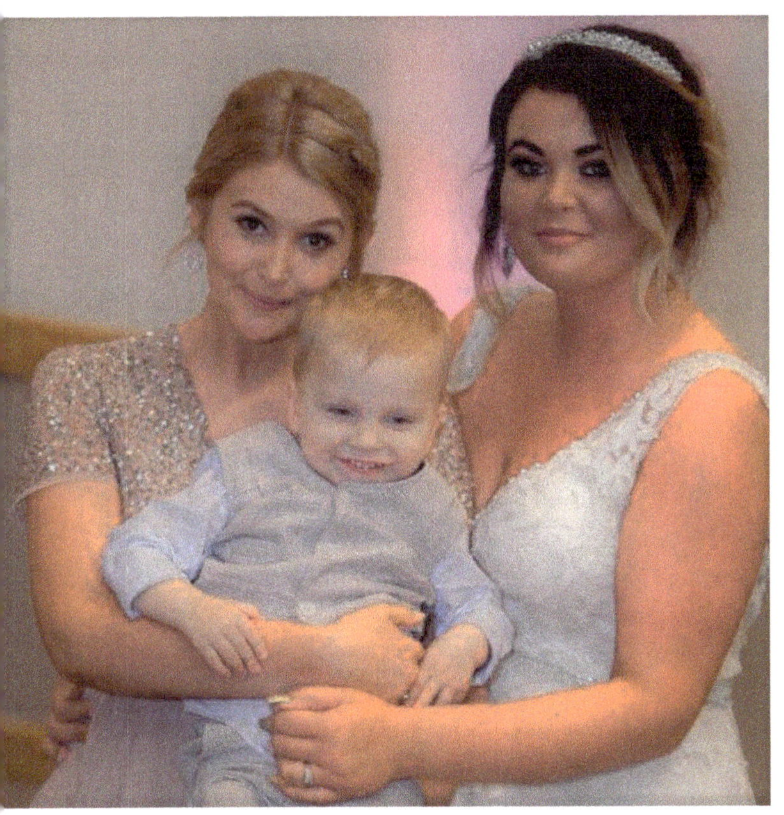

Left to right: May, William and Evie, at Evie's wedding

very beginning of my relationship with Mark. Of course, as children they didn't understand my fertility treatment, and nor should they have been expected to, but as soon as they were old enough to make sense of it all they became extremely supportive. I will always be grateful to them for this and I am incredibly proud of them. So, it's really important to me to make time for family gatherings, although we do see the girls on a regular basis. I think our first proper event as an extended family was William's christening, on May 28th, 2017, just before his first birthday. The church, St Mary Magdalene, is just around the corner from our house. After the ceremony, we had a party at home, where my friend Julie once again made herself indispensable, ensuring the guests had everything they needed, even though she was a guest herself. It was a lovely occasion, with an ideal combination of close friends and family celebrating the birth of our beautiful son. We had invited Dr Shehata, not just out of gratitude but because we like him very much too. Unfortunately, he couldn't make it, but he sent us a card with a lovely handwritten message, and a beautiful silver-plated Wedgwood keepsake box in the shape of a rabbit, which now holds William's first curl.

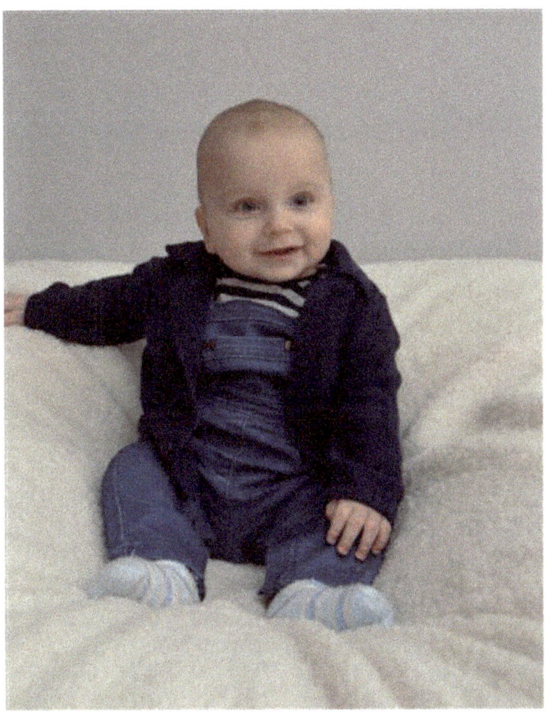

William

CHAPTER NINETEEN

Sometimes I wonder how Mark's and my relationship might have been without the turmoil of my many miscarriages. There's no point in pretending that it wouldn't have been any different, that our love for each other was so deep that it would have been unaffected by the fertility hell. Yes, our love was strong, and it still is, but it was certainly tested, over and over again.

Do I think that Mark might have been happier with someone else? Someone who either had children of her own already or was content with being a stepmother? This is something that has caused me considerable worry at times, and I don't mean in a jealous kind of way. It's just that when you love someone, their happiness is obviously important to you. I'm not miserable by nature, the opposite in fact, and hated it when my own deep unhappiness brought Mark down too.

I know that, sometimes, my sadness was almost a physical presence in our home. We could be laughing in front of a sitcom on a weekend, takeaway on our laps, and then the adverts would come on. There might be an advert, say, for a flash car – fine, I like cars. Then perhaps an advert for a chocolate bar – I like chocolate too. Then an advert for baby wipes, 'for the best baby skin in the world', and I'm floored. My food suddenly tastes like cardboard. I don't say anything, but Mark knows, and when the programme comes back on, his laughter is quieter. My unborn babies were everywhere, yet nowhere at all.

I've read about other couples who struggle to conceive and in some ways their experiences and feelings are similar to mine and Mark's. After repeated failure of conception, the romance of their relationship is replaced by science: charts, temperatures and diagrams take the place of kisses, cuddles and sometimes even joy itself. Performance becomes less about providing mutual satisfaction and more about reaching targets. The aim of conceiving a child takes precedence and the days of lovemaking 'just for fun' become a thing of the past. Obviously, this can put a strain on even the strongest relationship, with blame and recrimination creeping in like a poisonous gas.

Apart from a couple of occasions (my very first IVF and the first occasion in Prague), my initial fertility treatment was always successful, so Mark and I didn't really have the problems that these couples experience. But there was still hurt and anger, on both sides. My own hurt couldn't be blamed on Mark; it was simply one part of my natural feelings of loss. And my anger was mostly the result of frustration at my seemingly never-ending plight, although there were times when I was angry with myself for being unable to accept life without a child of my own.

For Mark, though, it was different – I was often the cause of his strong negative emotions, albeit unintentionally. It must have been pure hell for him at times, living with someone so focussed on having a baby but never able to achieve her heart's desire. I know that so often I was just not good company anymore. Being with someone who was either always crying or on the verge of it would have been enough to test anybody's patience.

One particular occasion when Mark lost his temper with me stays in my mind. It was a couple of days after another miscarriage – one of those times when I'd been kicked so hard that I could not get back up again. All I could do was lie on the sofa and cry. I had been crying all day, was still in my dressing-gown and hadn't even brushed my teeth. Although Mark never expected me to cook for him, I knew he would be hungry after work so I should at least chop some veg. But I couldn't move and was still lying there when he got home. I could see him taking in the dirty mugs and pile of clothes for washing that hadn't made it to the utility room. I could see him getting riled.

Then he just lost it – "There's more to life than lying around crying all the time, Louise!"

I wish his words had the effect of making me jump off the

sofa, into the shower, put on make-up and some funky clothes and say, "Come on then, let's go clubbing!", but it was as if I were paralysed, by hopelessness and grief. I shuddered as Mark slammed the door behind him, then lay my head back down on the cushion and cried even more.

So, during all my heartache, it was easy to forget that Mark was under intense strain too, that the loss was not mine alone. But, the more I miscarried, the more irrational my thoughts became. I admit that in my craziest moments I even began to think that Mark was pleased that I had miscarried. I never said this to him, but he probably guessed. The poor man – trying so hard to comfort me, and that's the thanks he gets!

Because I want my story to be completely honest, I feel it's important to say that there are times when I still struggle greatly. I suppose the reasons for this are very simple – trauma and grief. Although I don't like labels for people, it's pretty clear that, as in my GP's opinion, I'm suffering from post-traumatic stress disorder. Little analysis is needed to understand why. I know that to conquer PTSD is a long and difficult process (and can sometimes be impossible, no matter how much time and effort is put into it), and that professional help is almost always needed.

I feel a bit differently, though, about my ongoing grief. I have a higher level of acceptance of this and don't really see it as something that has to be challenged. Grief, after all, is natural and has no limits. Nobody has the right to say to another person, "Right, that's it, your time is up – you must stop grieving now." As long as I don't allow my feelings for all my unborn children to detract from the love I have for my son then the grieving process should ultimately be a positive one. I don't want to forget my miscarriages; I just want to reach a stage of accepting them. I think I'm almost there.

As I reflect on everything that has happened in my long quest for motherhood, I still feel pain for all my babies who never got to feel the sun on their skin and the earth beneath their feet. Who never got to hear me say to them, "I love you". But I reassure myself that even though I am a busy mum now with William, one day I will be an even busier mum, in heaven.

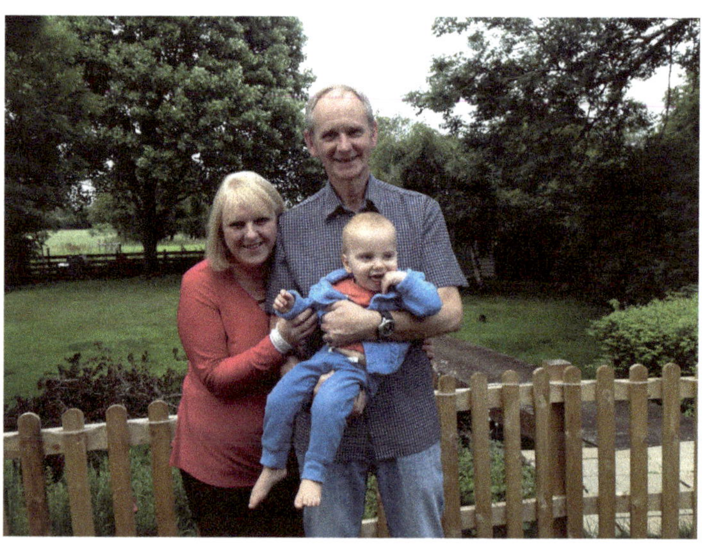

I would like to say a special thank you to:

Dad
My sister Julie and brother-in-law David
My stepdaughters May and Evie
Uncle Bob and Aunty Gayle
Uncle Ed and Aunty Norma
Aunty Carol and Uncle Ray
Butch
Ke Wang
Friends C. D., Julie Stevenson, Samantha Highley,
Clair Stewart, Liz Craig and Lisa Nichols
Dr Hassan Shehata and his PA Cheryl Estall
The staff at the Silver Star Unit of the John Radcliffe
Hospital
The Gynem Clinic in Prague, in particular Drs Milan
Mrázek and Tomas Rieger, and Patient Co-ordinator
Richard Kveck
Clare Pugh
My midwife Tracey Hatt
And, of course, Mark – for everything

Please contact me if you want further help or advice:
Email: babydreams@louisejwarneford

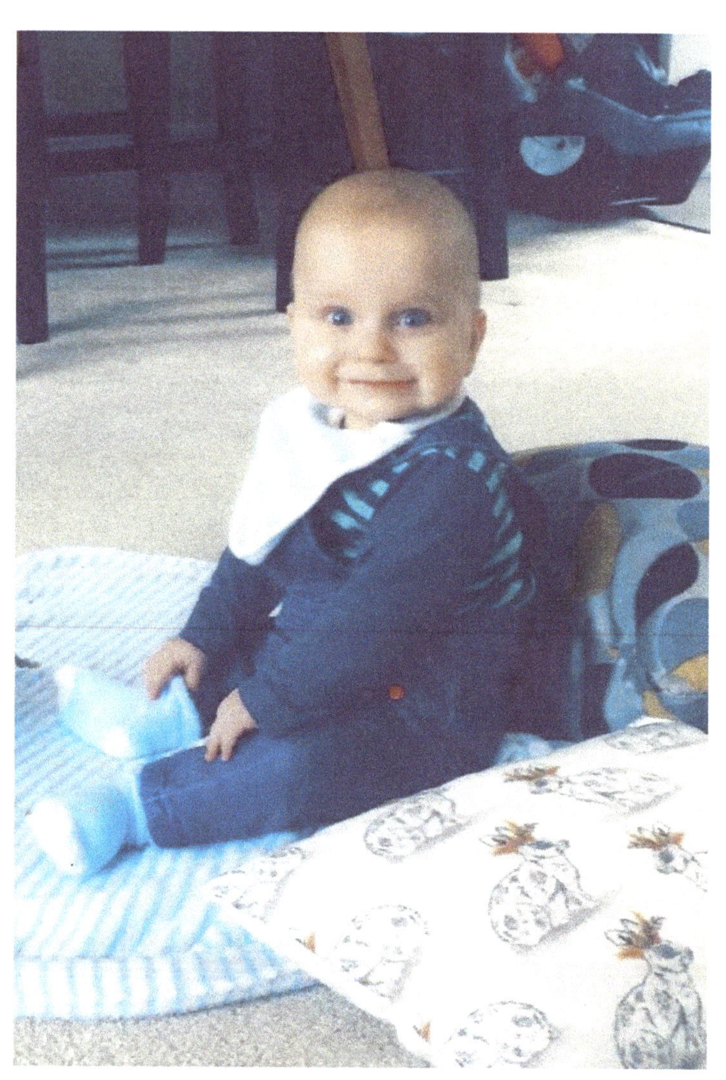

www.ingramcontent.com/pod-product-compliance
Lightning Source LLC
Chambersburg PA
CBHW060749240726

48664CB00009BA/1674